HEALTH CARE IN MOBILE:
AN ORAL HISTORY OF THE 1940S

Joy HP Harriman

ISBN: 1463575246
ISBN-13: 9781463575243

PREFACE

This book presents a small oral history of the delivery of health care in Mobile, Alabama, from the late 1930s to the early 1950s. It includes the beliefs, behaviors, expectations, and experiences of individuals whose lives have been entwined with community and health care: men and women from different cultures, social classes, and ethnic and racial groups whose differences and similarities combine to present their memories. Individually they are physicians and nurses, family members, an administrator, and a driver. Collectively they present common experiences that offer a glimpse of a very real health culture that has been mostly forgotten, as it existed before interstates, insurance, and intensive care units.

This isn't a history of professional or institutional medicine; it's a work of local health and medical history. Other books about health care during this time focus on scientific and technical aspects. Clearly it was a time of monumental growth. When these individuals were interviewed in the early 1990s, there were only a few books published about health care based on oral history. The spoken memories in this book are faithfully reproduced to allow you to understand the emotions, thoughts, perspective, culture, and assessment of the times. These narratives provide recollections about self and relationships with others that are seldom provided in such depth. That is their gift —coming to know each person's story as if you'd joined them at the dinner table.

What was life like living through these scientific breakthroughs and developments? Technological sophistication created a domino effect with repercussions in every aspect of daily life and the practice of health care. Caring for the health of a community has always required more than practicing objective scientific knowledge. It takes into account a wider range of elements and decision making.

The experiences shared here illustrate a changing spectrum of personal expectations about health concepts, therapeutics, and negotiation for power and resources in a culture affected by science, politics, economics, law, professional factors, gender, and social relationships.

These personal histories make important contributions. First, they remind us about the people, ideas, and events that preceded us. They offer a way to understand those organizations that created twenty-first-century medicine. Second, they show that these people were supported and troubled by features of modern medicine just as we are.

There are limitations in this account. Interviews with members of additional health care occupations—pharmacists, X-ray technicians, and anesthetists, for example—would have enriched the presentation. A broader scope including social class, ethnicity, or those from more rural areas would have added understanding. Unfortunately it wasn't possible to locate many people in this age group who fit these criteria.

The individuals chosen for this book met some not-so-scientific criteria: their experiences were in the time frame, and they were "alive, upright, and taking nourishment." They were smart, active, still had work to do and a purpose in their steps. They represented a range of socioeconomic and educational backgrounds. They wanted to be interviewed and signed the release consents for each edited interview as well as their personal photos. They have given permission for their real names and personal photos to be used in publications resulting from the interviews.

As the medical librarian of a large Southern hospital in Mobile, Alabama, I had the delicious opportunity of meeting vitally interesting people. Physicians, nurses, administrators, and visitors frequently passed through the medical library. Many came to request information and some just came to visit. Each had a story to tell and trusted me to ensure it got told.

Ten interviews are presented. Included are three women, seven men, one African American, nine whites, one ambulance driver and fireman, one administrator, two nurses, two wives, and five physicians. One was from Mississippi, one from New Orleans, five were originally from Mobile, nine had spent most of their lives in Mobile, one had lived all over the world, and two were from rural Alabama. They are all modest people, minimizing their accomplishments and involvements. Don't be fooled—each knew they were pioneers in a brand new world.

They were tape-recorded, transcribed, and edited only for readability or clarity. Interview recordings and transcripts have been donated to the University of South Alabama Archives and Museum in Mobile, Alabama. This book is organized chronologically based on the individual's birth year. The disadvantage of this choice is some overlap of topics among chapters. Arranging it in this manner helped me have a fuller view of the community.

Mobile Health Care Providers

Name	Birth date	Occupation	Professional training, graduation date	Practice location(s)	Age at time of interview
A. A. Wood	1905– 1999	surgeon	Springhill College, 1922 Tulane Medical School, 1931 Internship, City Hospital	Providence Hospital Private practice	89
Marguerite Wiggins Russell Franklin	1906– 2005	wife, James A Franklin, Sr.	Emerson Institute, 1924 Pratt University, Brooklyn, 1926 Lincoln University, Pennsylvania, 1911 Michigan University Medical School, 1915	Private practice	95
J.B. Foster	1907– 1995	ambulance driver	Mobile Fire Department, 1932 Fire Inspector and Investigator	City Hospital City Fire Department	87
E. G. DeBakey	1910– 2006	surgeon	Tulane Medical School, 1939 Internship, Charity Hospital, 1940 Residency, Washington University, St. Louis, Missouri, 1942 and 1948	Mobile Infirmary City Hospital Private practice	84

S.N. Rumpanos	1914– 2007	surgeon	University of Alabama, 1935 Duke University Medical School, 1937 Internship, City Hospital, Baltimore, Maryland Residency, University of Maryland, Baltimore, Maryland, City Hospital in Mobile, and US Navy Hospital in Bethesda	Mobile Infirmary City Hospital Private practice	80
H. N. Webster	1915– 2006	general practice	University of Alabama, 1937 Jefferson Medical College, 1941	Mobile Infirmary City Hospital ADDESCO Private practice	86
S. Eichold	1916– 2006	general practice	Tulane, 1936 Tulane Medical School, 1940 Internship, Touro, 1941 Residency City Hospital, Mobile	Mobile Infirmary City Hospital Private practice	84
A. W. Jerome	1918– 1999	nurse	Judson College, 1940 Touro Infirmary, 1932 Judson College, honorary PhD, 1993	Providence Hospital Private practice	77
E. C. Bramlett	1919– 2000	hospital administrator	University of Mississippi, 1940	Mobile Infirmary	75
M.W. Gatti	1925–	nurse manager operating room	Providence Hospital Nursing School, 1946	Providence Hospital Doctors Hospital	70

CHAPTER 1

This chapter introduces the hospitals of Mobile, Alabama, located centrally which was the pattern common to most Southern metropolitan areas. All five were located within a few blocks of each other, enabling white physicians, who crossed the boundaries of race, religion, and income in their practices, efficient access to the different accommodations their patients needed.

Before 1931, every year huge epidemics swept through American cities and carried away tens of thousands of people. There was nothing that anyone could do until the discovery of sulfa drugs (Hager). During the 1930s, the availability of medicines as we know them today was nil. Those who became patients first used their home knowledge of healing and folk medicine before calling for the doctor. Caring for patients was 80 percent hand holding and 20 percent medical knowledge because there wasn't much knowledge to be had. Even getting to the hospital was a gamble for those whose situation was bad enough to require admission. Hospitals were not the positive high-technology care centers they grew to become. During this time there was no air conditioning, most hospital materials were handmade and reusable, nurses were little more than watchful eyes and housekeepers, and all bills were paid by the patient—there was no such thing as insurance.

This chapter then moves to present the predominant issues encountered by the interviewees.

Mobile Hospitals

Geographically the five hospitals were located in Mobile

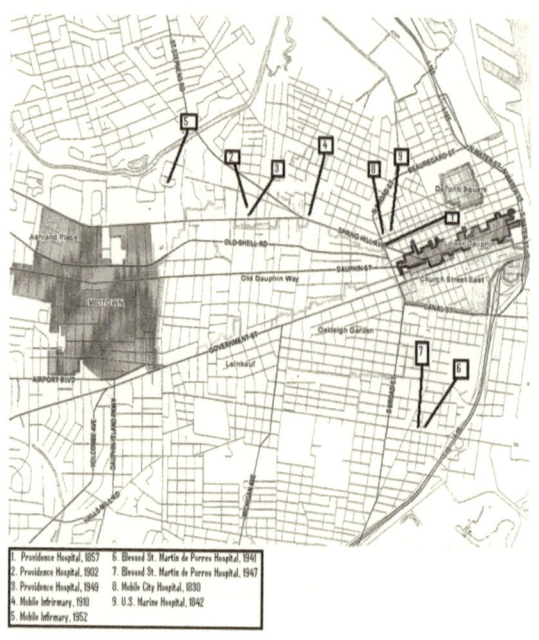

1. Providence Hospital, 1857	6. Blessed St. Martin de Porres Hospital, 1941
2. Providence Hospital, 1902	7. Blessed St. Martin de Porres Hospital, 1947
3. Providence Hospital, 1948	8. Mobile City Hospital, 1830
4. Mobile Infirmary, 1910	9. U.S. Marine Hospital, 1842
5. Mobile Infirmary, 1952	

Providence Hospital

The first Providence Hospital (1, map) was bounded by St. Anthony, Broad, Jefferson, and St. Louis Streets. The land was purchased in 1854 and a year later the completed two-and-a-half-story, 60-bed hospital was known as the Providence Infirmary. In 1857, the *Mobile Daily Register* read, "The first floor is devoted to male patients, the second to females, and servants are accommodated in the spacious airy attic. From front to rear, and from the East end, the public wards, a spacious passage admits the free circulation of air from every quarter. In the rear, and on each side, are large grounds and gardens for exercise and unlimited ventilation. Cleanliness in every place and of everything is more marked than in the neatest dwelling."

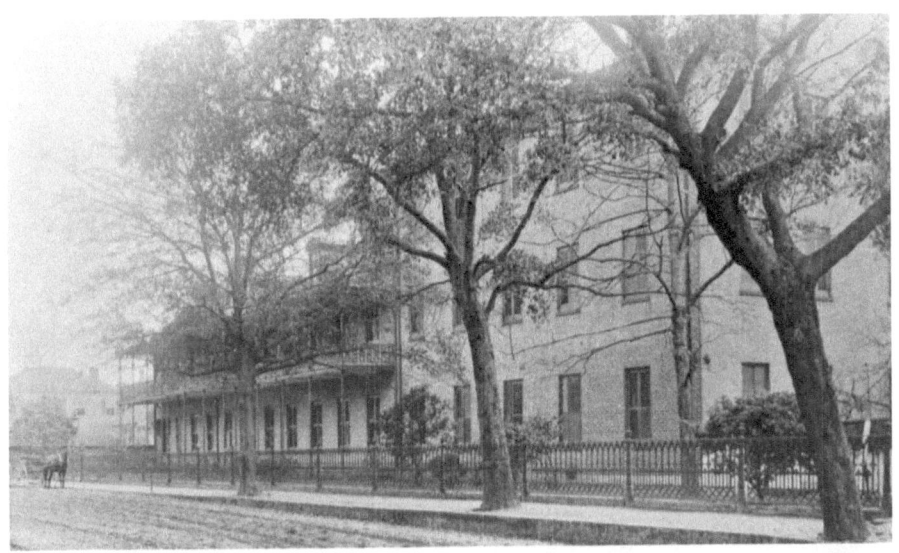

Providence Infirmary (1857), bounded by St. Anthony, Broad, Jefferson, and St. Louis Streets (Courtesy of the Daughters of Charity Archives – Evansville, IN)

By 1901 both the Providence and City Hospitals boasted modern operating rooms, although until the 1950s windows in all surgical suites were thrown open to catch whatever breezes might have been available.

As Mobile grew, a larger hospital was needed. In 1902 at 1504 Spring Hill Avenue (2, map) the second Providence Hospital, a Mediterranean-inspired stucco building, opened. An east wing was added in 1908, but the hospital remained largely unchanged until 1950. That year the population of Mobile was 230,000, and Providence Hospital contained only one hundred beds.

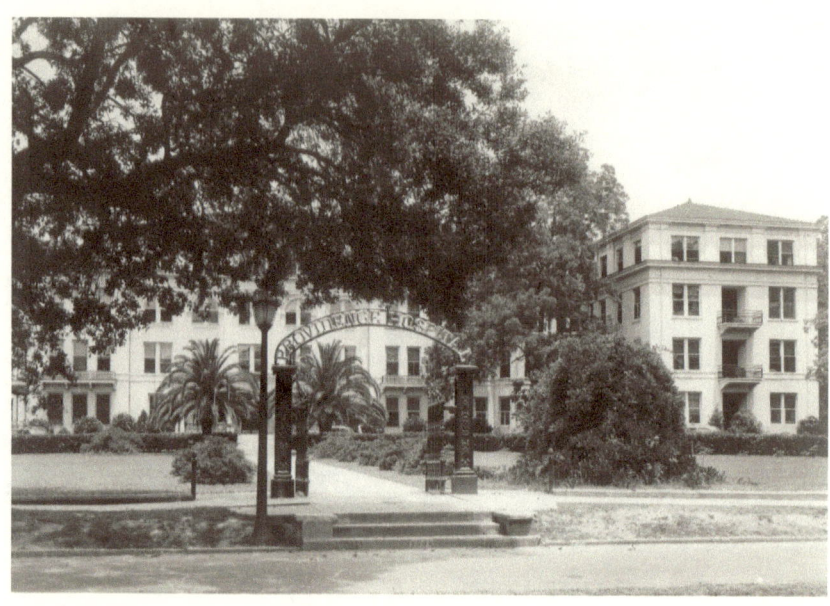

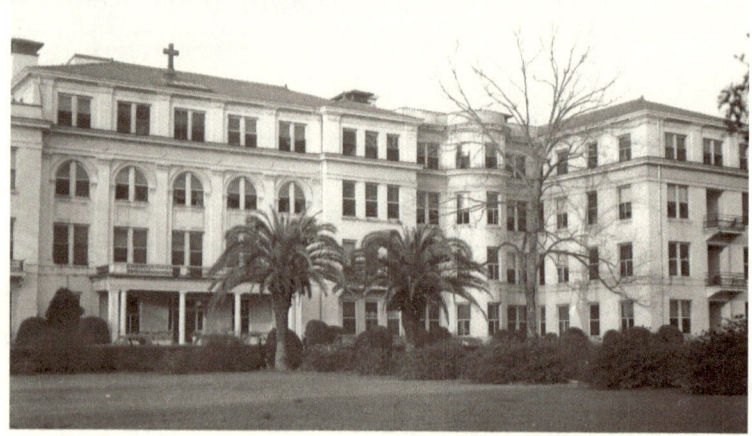

Providence Hospital, built in 1902, 1504 Spring Hill Avenue (Courtesy of the Daughters of Charity Archives – Evansville, IN)

By 1919 hospital rates had risen to five dollars per day, and a typical maternity stay would total 33 dollars, including meals, medicine, and lab tests. Operating rooms early in the century became busier as surgical techniques for the treatment of disease became more common. The operating room record book from the 1930s lists the occasional bullet removal, but the most frequently performed procedures were appendectomies and tonsillectomies. Delivery costs would triple by the 1940s, when the care for delivering a baby, including bracelet and birth certificate, cost 116 dollars.

The ground was broken for the third Providence Hospital in February 1949 (3, map) on land immediately in front of the second hospital on Springhill Avenue. The entire patient population was moved in April 1950 to the Allen Memorial Home beside the hospital property and stayed there until August 1952, when the new hospital admitted its first patient. The new facility cost four million dollars, was eight stories, and held 250 beds. Two of the hospital's features that created headlines at the time were the fact that it was completely air-conditioned and had fluorescent lighting.

Soon after the second Providence Hospital was built, the Daughters of Charity saw the need to train nurses, opening the school of nursing in 1902, the first such school in Mobile and the second in Alabama. The first class had two students graduating in 1905. The training was far from easy. Annie Mae Wainwright, class of 1911, wrote, "The girls maintained a 12-hour day during their three years of training with only a half hour off for their meals. They received only a half day off a week." The students were housed on the fourth floor of the hospital. A nurses' home adjacent on Catherine Street was completed in December 1940.

In 1982 the Daughters designed a futuristic hospital on a 250-acre campus west of town. The sixty-million-dollar facility accepted its first patients in July 1987.

The Mobile Infirmary

In 1909, a group of Mobile women established an infirmary and a school of nursing. Though their husbands managed the money as trustees, the women organized and ran the effort. In October 1910, the first hospital building of the Mobile Infirmary (4, map) was opened, containing 34 paying wards and two free wards, with four beds in each. There were also two wards with four beds in each for one dollar per day, operating rooms, and one laboratory. It was located at what was known as Five Points, the intersections of Springhill, Ann, and St. Stephens Streets.

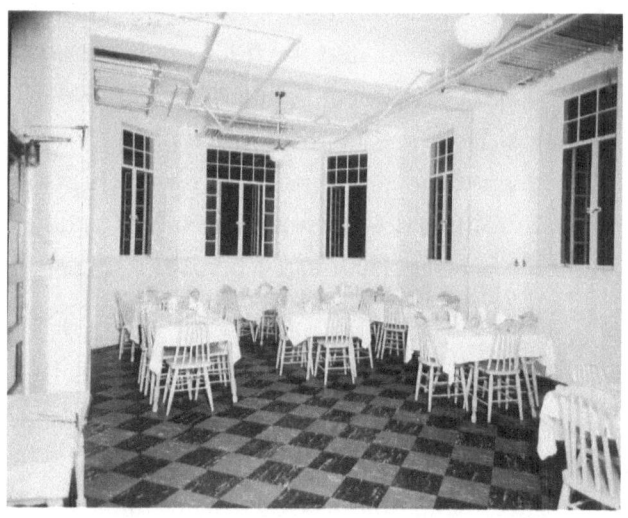

Cafeteria in the Mobile Infirmary (1910) (Courtesy Mr. E.C. Bramlett, Sr.)

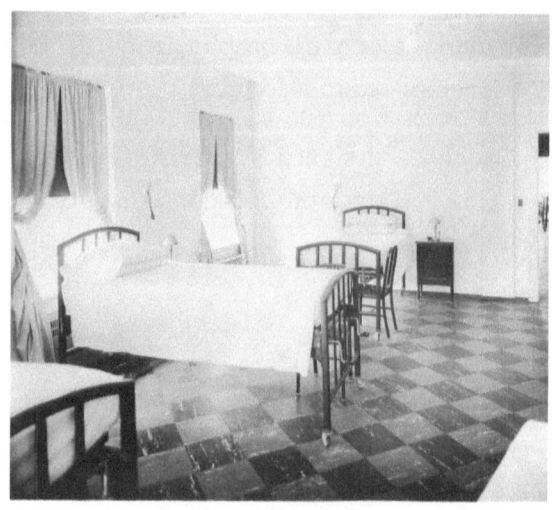

Mobile Infirmary hospital room (1910) (Courtesy Mr. E.C. Bramlett, Sr.)

The first class of the Mobile Infirmary School of Nursing was also admitted. One of the first four graduates in 1913 was Katherine White-Spunner, who returned to Mobile in 1933 to become the Mobile Infirmary's superintendent.

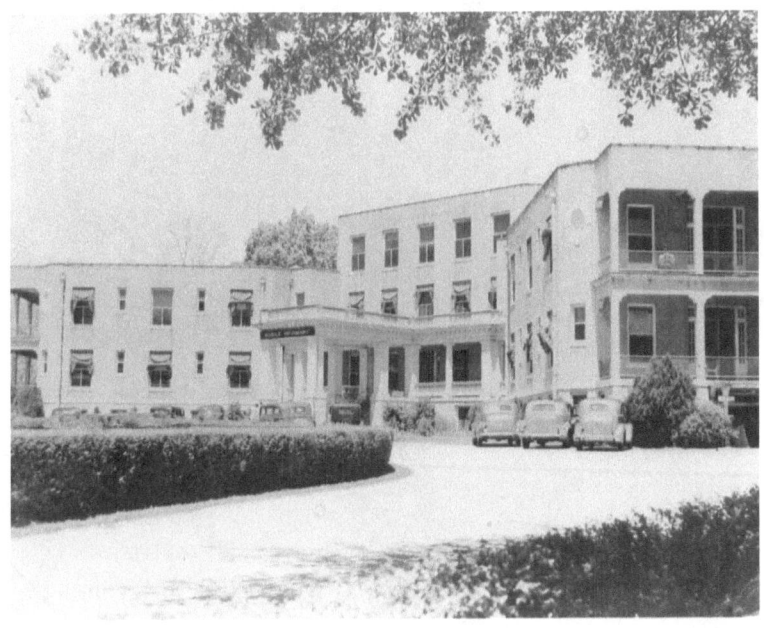

Mobile Infirmary side view (1910) (Courtesy Mr. E.C. Bramlett, Sr.)

During the next 42 years, more wards and wings were added, but by 1946, the 150 hospital beds did not adequately serve a severely overburdened postwar Mobile. Some 28 Protestant, Jewish, and Greek ministers of Mobile joined a campaign for a new Mobile Infirmary. On Sunday, June 8, 1947, all town ministers exchanged pulpits to speak with one voice to Mobile congregations about the need for a new hospital. The next day, half of the two million dollars needed to build the new Infirmary was pledged by these congregations.

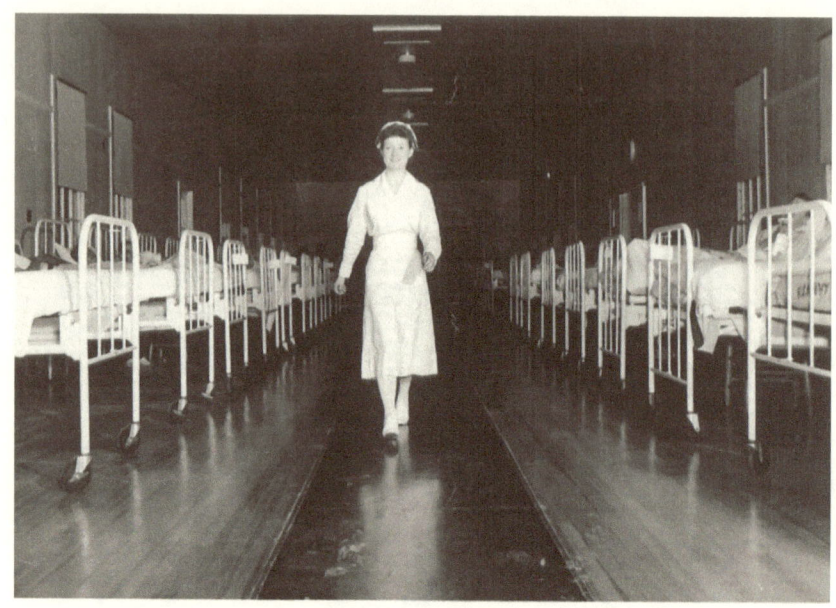

Mobile Infirmary nurse (1944)(Courtesy Mr. E.C. Bramlett, Sr.)

To assist with the new hospital, Mobile was allocated one of 33 top priorities for construction of new general hospital facilities under a state-wide master hospital plan. In allocating a top priority to Mobile for general hospital facilities, the state of Alabama had stipulated that the institution must participate in internship for medical students and extend nurses' training courses.

Alabama was also one of the top five states to receive federal funds allocated under the Hill-Burton Act (1946). The state stood to be the fifth-greatest recipient, receiving fifteen million dollars in federal aid hospital funds during the next five years under the act. Mobile received allocations totaling five hundred thousand dollars to two Mobile hospitals for new buildings under the Hill-Burton Act. The Mobile Infirmary was allocated three hundred thousand dollars and Providence Hospital two hundred thousand dollars.

The second Mobile Infirmary (5, map) opened in 1952 with 285 beds. It grew to 704 beds in 1985, making the Infirmary Alabama's largest non-government hospital.

Blessed St. Martin de Porres Hospital

The first Blessed St. Martin de Porres Hospital (1941) (6, map) was located at 623 S. Wilkinson Street and cared for black maternity patients. It was a Catholic hospital, owned and operated by the Sisters of Mercy, but 85 percent of the patients were non-Catholic. The hospital consisted of one ward of five beds, a delivery room, a nursery, an office, and a kitchen. At that time there were only four beds available in Mobile for black maternity patients. In 1942, another ward was added, bringing the total beds to nine. Despite a lack of modern conveniences or equipment, the care provided brought remarkable results: over 2500 babies were born with only three maternal deaths. All complicated cases and those requiring surgery were transferred to City Hospital.

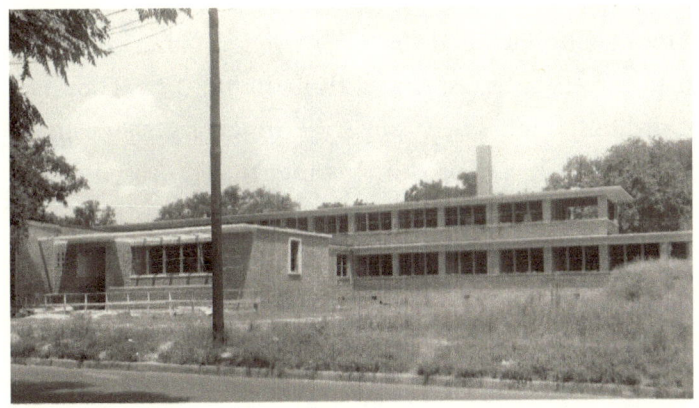

Martin de Porres Hospital, built in 1941, at 623 S. Wilkinson Street Prior to the 1950s, black doctors in Mobile didn't have access to the city's hospitals, so they treated patients either at home or at infirmaries set up by private physicians. The facilities weren't good, but they were the best that could be had at the time. The situation changed with the opening of St. Martin de Porres Hospital.

A state Department of Health survey revealed that only 34 percent of the beds needed for the care of blacks were available. Realizing that need and intending to give greater opportunities to black physicians to practice medicine, Bishop Toolen spearheaded an effort to build a new hospital. In 1947 ground was broken for the new hospital in the Choctaw City Park located at Virginia Street and South Washington Avenue (7, map). Hill-Burton funds were approved and construction started in February 1949. Opening in April 1950, the hospital bed capacity was 35, with two private rooms, eight semiprivate, and three wards of four beds each.

The black community contributed furnishings, especially for the pediatric ward, solarium, and waiting rooms, as well as necessary clinical equipment. The hospital had a biracial staff of eight Sisters, five black graduate nurses, 12 practical nurses and aides, and one black X-ray technician. The medical staff of the hospital was also biracial, one of the few of its kind in the South. With the advent of integration, the hospital closed in 1971.

Mobile City Hospital

The Mobile City Hospital (8, map) was located at the northeast corner of Broad Street, at St. Anthony. Built in 1830 by Thomas S. James, Mobile's third hospital has been preserved in its original design except for additions at each end, serving without interruption through fires, yellow fever epidemics, and war. For 83 years, between 1861 and 1959, it was administered by the Sisters of Charity.

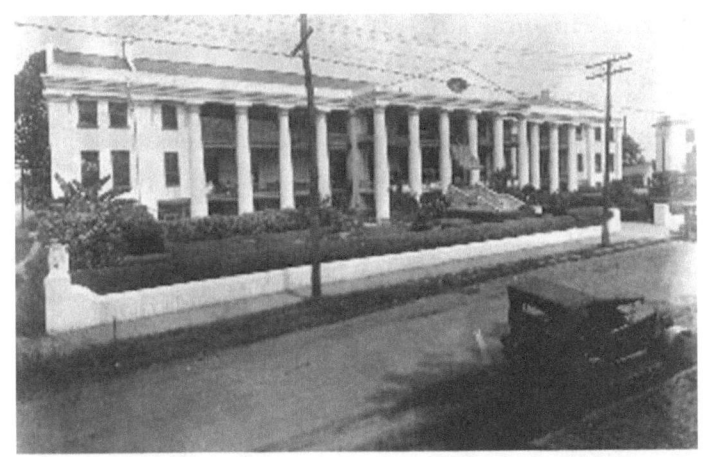

Mobile City Hospital

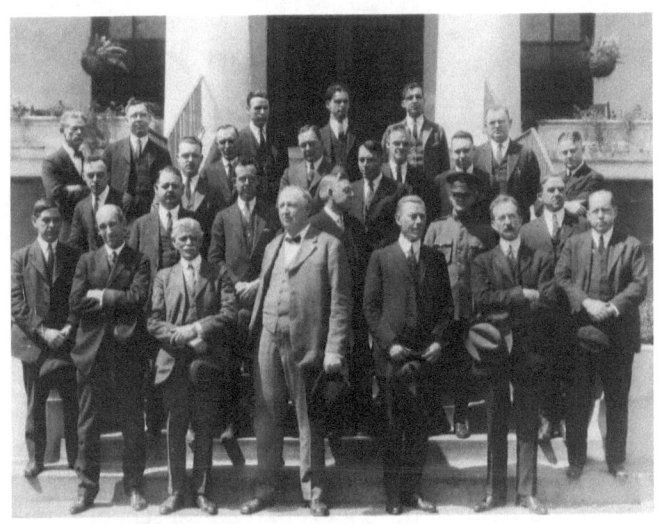

City Hospital medical staff photo (1922) From Dr. S. Rumpanos: "There was . . .
old man Acker. He thought he was the king because he used to be a teacher at the
old medical school when it was here in Mobile. And he and Dr. Purdue were the
biggest rivals you've ever seen. There was a picture of the Hospital staff and they're
standing with their backs to each other. They wouldn't even look at {each other}.
They got jealous of each other."

U.S. Marine Hospital

The U.S. Marine Hospital (9, map) (Mobile County Health Department) was a government hospital for merchant marine seamen. It is located at the northwest corner of St. Anthony at Jefferson. Built in 1838 to 1841, it was in operation from 1842 to 1952, having served both Confederate and Union troops from 1861 to 1865.

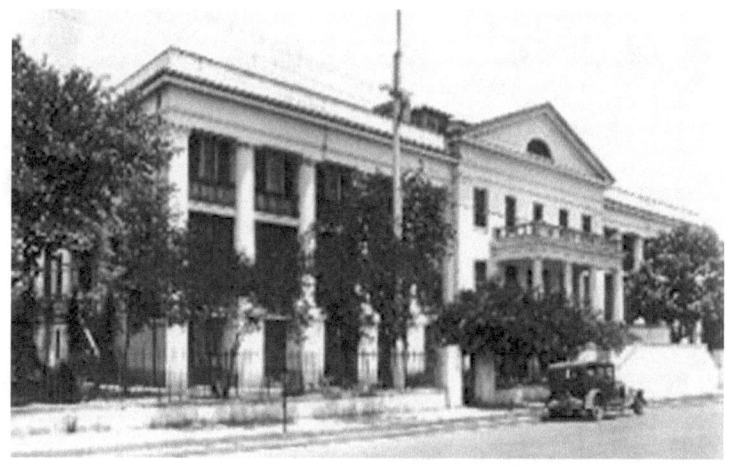

US Marine Hospital was sometimes referred to as the tuberculosis sanitarium

Discrimination in Medical School

Social and racial changes in the US have always affected the delivery of health care. Anti-Semitism of the 1930s in medical school admissions gave way and was later replaced with racism and integration of medical staffs in the 1950s and 1960s. American medical schools have been a battleground in the struggle for civil rights and the discrimination has never been restricted to one group. Jews and Catholics have experienced difficulties in getting into the medical profession. For Catholics, the problem was manageable, since their own schools and hospitals guaranteed them access to medical training and clinical experience. Jews saw little discrimination in medicine prior to about 1920, but the next 30 years saw both official and unofficial discrimination against Jewish applicants to medical schools.

Documentation of discrimination is difficult. The subject was touchy and many academic institutions denied its existence. However, quotas were placed on Jews in order to maintain what school administrators felt was a proper proportionate balance within the student body. Particularly acute in medicine, discrimination against Jewish students continued at all college levels during the 1930s.

As long as medical schools vied with each other for students, white males had little difficulty in gaining acceptance. In the early 1900s Jews constituted a relatively small percentage of the population and presented no economic threat to practicing physicians. Following the Flexner Report in 1910, standards for medical education tightened and the number of US medical schools was gradually reduced from 137 (1910) to 76 (1931).

By the 1920s, the factors affecting medical school selection had changed. The efforts of organized medicine to raise educational standards and to limit entrance into the profession greatly reduced the number of available places for medical students. At the same time, the children of the massive wave of Russian Jewish immigrants who had entered America around the turn of the century were beginning to move into the professions. Fully 50 percent of the nearly fourteen thousand men and women attempting to matriculate in 1920 were Jewish. Of the six thousand accepted, however, only 17 percent were Jewish (Lazarus, 22). It was also disproportionately difficult for a Jew to get into any other profession or most good colleges. A Jew could not stay in many hotels, buy real estate in many places, get a job in many firms, or enter a club as a guest, let alone as a member.

At Harvard College in 1922, President A. Lawrence Lowell suggested a quota system for Jewish applicants, which resulted in much faculty dissension. A separate school, the Harvard Medical School did not establish a fixed number, but historians have acknowledged that anti-Semitism was a significant factor in the low "incidence" of Jewish students there from 1910 to 1935 (Beecher, 483).

A second standards tightening occurred in 1933 at the recommendation of the American Medical Association (AMA) in response to the declining incomes of physicians during the Depression. Denied access elsewhere, 65 percent of 1,802 refugee medical practitioners were concentrated in New York City in 1943, adding to the competition. Dr. Shepard Jerome, husband to Annelle Jerome, was one Jewish student accepted into Harvard College. She was a devout Baptist from the Alabama countryside and he was originally an Orthodox Jew who had experienced the harsh anti-Semitism at Harvard Medical School. He hadn't told her his background because, as she recounted, "this was when the Jews were so unpopular. He had been ostracized the whole time he was growing up because he was Jewish. Anti-Semitism was strong, very much so, especially up in lower Massachusetts, in Boston, where he was raised."

Since Jews were concentrated in the northeastern cities, policies which restricted the number of admissions from large cities, geographic areas, or out of state all served to keep the number of Jewish medical students to a minimum. School officials claimed no anti-Semitism, but argued that a disproportionate number of Jews in medicine and law would breed resentment. Thus the quota system was in the best interest of the Jews (Duffy, 288). One side of the argument held that the country had too many Jewish medical students and that the "racial imbalance" should be corrected. The other side saw this as anti-Semitic discrimination and vigorously fought restrictions against admission of Jewish applicants (Sokoloff, 497 and 299). These ethnic prejudices have been replaced with open-admission practices.

Medicines

As late as the 1920s, there were only about a dozen drugs that reliably worked. The use of pharmaceuticals was not part of medical care. Up until the 1930s, research to develop new drugs generally failed to achieve very much (Rothstein, 122; Stevens, 597). Almost all prescription drugs were "generic," referred to as "standard drugs." They were not marketed, but were sold by salesmen armed with price lists to those pharmacies who did not compound their own standard preparations (Redwood, 249).

This was changed as a result of the "wonder drug" era, which started with the first sulfanilamide (an antistreptococcal), synthesized in Germany in 1932 and launched by Bayer in 1935 under the brand name Prontosil (Duffy, 296; Bordley, 447). The revolutionary feature of the sulfa drugs was that they operated on an entirely new principle: instead of killing the bacteria, they interfered with the growth and reproduction cycle of the microbes, rendering them harmless. It was miraculous in that for the first time in history physicians could effectively treat a range of common diseases.

During the 1930s, Dr. Sam Eichold drove the car for Dr. P. D. McGehee (Tiny) in Mobile and would help as he could. He assisted when there were no antibiotics for treatment and home visits were the norm. "We had no antibiotics. We had no therapeutic modalities. The medicines we used were Prontosil—a red liquid for infections—and that was the *only* thing we had. This was pre–sulfa drugs, maybe 1935–1936. Dr. Doehring brought it from Germany [to Mobile]. It was a liquid, it was injectable. Later, after World War II we had sulfanilamide, sulfadiazine, and sulfathiazole."

Similarly, during the 1940s penicillin was made available to the American public. There was stunned wonderment in the voices of those witnessing penicillin's results. Annelle Jerome was a nurse at Tulane Infirmary in New Orleans in 1942. Her recollection of the introduction of penicillin seems overly dramatic, until realizing that during those years death would as easily come from a bad cold as from a heart attack. "I was the very first nurse at Tulane Infirmary to give a shot of penicillin in 1942 in a pediatric ward to a child about ten years old. A miracle happened. It helped her and she overcame her illness. Immediately. It just looked like a miracle." Beginning with the discovery of the sulfa drugs in 1935 and until the middle of the 1950s, the mortality from childhood diseases, worldwide, went down by 90 percent. This was a turning point in human history, as the average lifespan for Americans was increased by more than ten years (Hager).

Contributing to the turning point was the ability to manufacture on a large scale. Penicillin was discovered in 1928, but it was not until World War II, with the huge increase in research, that penicillin was actually developed. For this the military entered into collaboration with academia and industry, achieving unprecedented levels of innovation (Hoyt, 38). Bordley comments, "Commercial firms already working on the production problem found they could step it up from one-liter bottles to *fifteen-thousand-gallon tanks*" (emphasis added) (Bordley, 357). The development of penicillin provides a striking illustration of the effectiveness of a well-financed and coordinated approach to the practical application of a basic medical discovery. No private, uncoordinated effort could have secured such results in a comparable period of time. With the exception of the atomic bomb project, the penicillin program had the highest priority of any military item during the war (Ginn, 144).

Following the penicillin program a cascade of new antibiotics and new drugs began, transforming the market for prescription drugs. The introduction of the sulfonamides in the late 1930s and the antibiotics and other drugs in the 1940s changed the world significantly by giving physicians, for the first time, a powerful weapon against disease (Stevens, 597). In the 1940s alone, wartime programs contributed to the development of new or significantly improved vaccines for ten of the 28 vaccine-preventable diseases identified in the twentieth century (Hoyt, 38).

While developing medicines, the United States also introduced the use of biological warfare. Dr. Socrates Rumpanos had entered the Navy in 1941 with full intention of going to the war. But the Navy put him back in school for 12 months. He was in the first group studying and creating biological warfare at Camp Detrick in Maryland in one of the most secret and work-intensive programs of World War II. After the war and having lived in an advanced scientific program for years, Dr. Rumpanos returned to Mobile, essentially stepping back into the late 1930s.

Ambulance Services

Getting to the hospital during this time could be as dangerous as being in a hospital. Frequently the early "ambulance" drivers were morticians from the funeral homes. They commonly provided emergency transportation because they were the only business in town with vehicles that could transport a person horizontally (O'Brien, 103; Smith and Holmes, 86). In many cities and towns, including Mobile, the community fire department provided a driver in support of the local hospital. Even in the 1950s and 1960s, many rural communities didn't have ambulance service and used the funeral home's hearse to have family taken to the hospital (Galdston, 510).

Initially, many attempted to meet their own medical needs, primarily using home remedies (Galdston, 510). They feared and avoided hospitalization, as the mortality rate of hospital-treated illnesses far exceeded that of illnesses treated at home. Mr. James B. "Red" Foster was a part-time ambulance driver for Mobile City Hospital starting in 1932. He was well known to physicians who interned in Mobile and were regular riders with him in the ambulance. His story is included for several reasons: because of his knowledge of the City Hospital and because his awareness of the practice and results of home remedies was firsthand. He frequently picked up patients who had used up their home remedy skills and couldn't get well. Going to a hospital, he knew, meant embracing the very real possibility of death.

When "Red" Foster became an ambulance driver "the skill of driving was not as well developed or universal as it is today" (Ginn, 41). The drivers were congenial, dedicated, helpful men who drove carefully and, when necessary, daringly, at a relatively fast speed" (Galdston, 510). Generally, ambulances were given all possible rights of way.

Insurance

As in all communities, Mobile had changing expectations of health care that moved from traditional reliance on home care to increasing dependence on professional institutional care. Patients moved from the norm of "call the doctor to come" to "get an appointment to go." The community expected better health care and over time that expectation changed medical care from a luxury to a necessity. This time frame also saw the introduction of a new kind of health care financing—insurance.

By 1930, the United States had as many or more medical, nursing, and dental schools and hospital beds per unit of population as it has today. However, many Americans had trouble paying for the medical care they needed. Between 1929 and 1930, average hospital receipts dropped from more than two hundred dollars per patient to less than 60 dollars. Occupancy rates continued to fall into the 1930s. Hospitals then began to consider insurance plans as a way to guarantee a steady cash flow, spreading the financial risk (Wasley, 11).

Locally based prepaid hospital plans began in several cities during the 1930s, most following the first plan conceived at Baylor (Dallas) in 1929. In return for a small monthly fee, the subscriber gained the promise of so many days of hospitalization per year along with discounts on special services, such as X-rays. This idea spread quickly, and multihospital insurance plans began sprouting up around the country, operating as not-for-profit organizations whose members were not exclusive to a single organization or occupation (H&HN, 13). The prepaid plan guaranteed both hospitals and doctors a source of income in uncertain times. Soon, many local plans were adding coverage for dependents and maternity care (Asplund, 7).

Then groups of nonprofit hospitals in several cities organized multiple-hospital insurance plans. These plans gave patients a choice of medical care providers, which attracted more patients, strengthening the income to the participating hospitals. This multiple-hospital plan served as a model for Blue Cross, established in 1932. These hospital plans changed the concept of insurance and forever changed the American health care system. The primary purpose of these plans, unlike other forms of insurance, was not to protect consumers from large, unforeseen expenses, but rather to keep hospitals in business by guaranteeing them a regular income. They helped to boost demand for hospital services and to stabilize hospital income streams, and they benefited consumers by giving them a predictable method of paying for their medical care (Wasley, 13).

They also provided prepaid coverage for physician services. Blue Cross and Blue Shield (BC/BS) plans grew despite the strong opposition of many physicians, who viewed prepaid benefits as a potential threat to their professional independence. The Medical Society of Mobile County held many meetings to discuss the merits of BC/BS coverage. Dr. Socrates Rumpanos recalled, "We tried to get set fees because Blue Cross asked us to, but we couldn't get physicians to agree. I asked them, begged them." Dr. Sam Eichold commented, "The mistake we made was we let Blue Cross Blue Shield write the contract and we had to agree to service the contract. And when they wrote the contract the doctors couldn't get together enough and say this stuff doesn't service our patients. We could have told them that we can't accept this. Instead we got stuck, because the doctors wouldn't get together."

A strong contribution made by BC/BS was the reimbursement procedure they adopted. This procedure, known as a cost-plus, was adopted by other insurance companies in order to compete and was also used by the Medicare program. Cost-plus allowed physicians to be reimbursed according to "reasonable and customary" charges, and hospitals were reimbursed on a percentage of their cost plus a percentage of their working and equity capital. This system permitted doctors to charge what they wanted, knowing they would be reimbursed, and created a perverse incentive for hospitals to increase costs because that meant increased income. Prior to World War II the patient was responsible for paying the hospital bill, and this had a restraining effect on hospital costs. The patient then wanted to get out of the hospital as soon as possible to save expenses. Now, with a third party paying the bill, the patient didn't object to being hospitalized, and when admitted, was in no hurry to be discharged (Wasley, 13).

Dr. Ernest G. DeBakey commented, "But the interesting thing about our time was that the patient was responsible for the insurance and for paying us. The patient paid us and the insurance paid the patient. And that's the way it should be now. See, I think the problem started when the doctor accepted the payments from the insurance company and relieved the patient of any responsibility. But they did that because they knew they were going to get paid. They were more interested in that than they were anything else."

The Social Security Act was signed in August 1935. Over the course of the next seven decades, it became one of the most influential, far-reaching health-related acts of Congress in the history of the US, eventually serving as the legislative launching pad for both Medicare and Medicaid (Gerber, 12).

In the 1940s, private insurance expanded rapidly as businesses began to use health benefits to get around wartime wage caps. Wartime wage and price controls prohibited employers from increasing salaries to attract workers; employer-provided health insurance was used as a bargaining chip to attract and retain workers. In 1942 the War Labor Board decided that fringe benefits up to 5 percent of wages would not be considered inflationary.

Total enrollment in group hospital plans grew from less than seven million to about twenty-six million subscribers from 1942 to 1945 (Wasley, 12). By 1949, employee benefit programs in collective bargaining agreements became widespread (Scofea, 3). During the war, labor unions were successful in negotiating hospital insurance for workers. Twenty-four percent of people in the US had hospital insurance in 1945, and by 1950 this number jumped to 50 percent (Dawley, 89).

An example of the move to accept hospital care by community members is seen in the use of hospital birthing services. In 1943, faced with an increase in young servicemen's families who did not have the financial means to purchase adequate pregnancy-related care, the federal government instituted the Emergency Maternity and Infant Care Program (EMIC). Before the program ended in 1946, over a million women and infants who received care under EMIC experienced the benefits of health insurance, and many who might have delivered at home were introduced to hospital obstetric care (Dawley, 89). The popularity of the hospital as the preferred place in which to give birth is seen in the increase of births in hospitals from 708,889 (1931) to 1,670,599 (1942) (H&HN, 12).

World War II Years and the Wartime Transformation of Mobile

Issues faced by those interviewed in this book included the changing of graduate medical education, the advent of insurance, and the necessity of and training of more specialized practitioners in medicine. But the phenomenal growth and transformation Mobile witnessed during the war had an equal impact on the whole community. During World War II Mobile was transformed into a major center of defense industry in the country. Once a sleepy port, Mobile's growth was rapid, unplanned and chaotic. In 1930 the county population was 118,363. By 1950 the county population had grown to 231,105.

Because Mobile was already an important railroad hub and port city, in 1940 the Army Air Corps chose it for the construction of Brookley Field west of Mobile. The facility modified B-24s and served as a military depot. By 1943 Brookley employed seventeen thousand civilians. The two largest shipyards employed more than forty thousand workers during the war. Alabama Dry Dock (ADDSCO) expanded its labor force from about one thousand in the late 1930s to nearly thirty thousand in the early 1940s. The Gulf Shipbuilding Corporation began production in 1940 and had more than ten thousand employees by the end of 1942. By 1943 the two largest firms, ADDSCO and Gulf Shipbuilding, employed forty thousand and were producing on average a ship each week.

The Census Bureau estimated that eighty-nine thousand people came to Mobile County between April 1940 and March 1943, changing the area fundamentally (Wikipedia). Many reports documented the inadequate housing and health care, the food shortages, the traffic congestion, the over-crowded schools, the near complete lack of recreational facilities, and the highest rate of increase in the cost of living in the nation (Nelson, 956). The population of the metropolitan area increased 75 percent from 1940 to 1944, making it the most congested urban area in the United States (Harrison, 276).

World War II's impact also launched the modern civil rights move-ments and forever changed the racial relations of the archetypical "South." Nowhere in the country did the war more disrupt established racial patterns as blacks and whites streamed into Mobile from the rural areas of Alabama, Mississippi, and west Florida (McLaurin, 47). The city's black population rose from 29,046 in 1940 to 45,819 in 1950, with nearly all of the increase occurring the war years (Loftin, 274). Mobile was unique in that three of its citizens achieved statewide prominence in Alabama's postwar effort to cope with changing patterns of race relations. John L. LeFlore was a postal clerk and executive secretary of the local chapter of the National Association for the Advancement of Colored People (NAACP), attorney Gessner McCorvey was chairman of the State Democratic Executive Committee and supported the state's conservatives on both racial and economic issues, and Senator Joseph N. Langan was a supporter of the policies of the National Democratic Party (Nelson, 963).

During the war, the combined efforts of LeFlore, McCorvey, and Langan saw black welders hired on an equal basis with whites by the shipyards. Whites at the Alabama Dry Docks and Shipbuilding Company rioted for two days in May 1943 because the Fair Employment Practices Commission had persuaded the company to upgrade 12 blacks to welding jobs. The 12 men worked an entire shift without incident, in a segregated gang where they attracted little attention. The next morning, however, the rumors began to fly (Nelson, 978). Later it was called "perhaps the single most dramatic conflict brought by wartime changes in the southern political economy" (Jones, 299). The rioting white workers used "pipes, clubs, and other weapons to drive black workers from . . . their jobs" (Jones, 299). Some blacks sustained serious injuries and virtually all of them experienced hours of terror, which ended only when United States Army troops from nearby Brookley Field arrived on Pinto Island to restore order (Nelson, 952; Loftin, 293).

During the war years, Mobile also saw a severe shortage of doctors and hospital facilities. The entire nation faced a shortage of doctors because fifty thousand of the country's approximately 185,000 doctors were in the armed forces. In the US, one doctor for every 1,500 people was regarded as a safe minimum standard. As of June 1, 1943, Alabama had one doctor for every 2,671 people. The number of physicians practicing in Mobile fell from 116 in 1940 to just 85 during wartime. Mobile County had only four midwives. The doubling of the city's population left housing and sanitation facilities overwhelmed and caused health problems that put Mobile in the national spotlight.

Dr. Harry Webster was the shipyard physician in Mobile. "We had a little hospital over there and I had about 30 patients over there at the time. It was a pretty good size when they were building as many ships as they built over there. It was a big business. As a matter of fact, by the time I had been at the docks about six or eight months and the state Public Health Service came to review over there and said you've got to have help, boy. I said I sure do, so they sent me some help ... They'd do that rather than to be shipped over to get shot at. So suddenly I had help."

The critical shortage of hospital facilities in Mobile was obvious as early as September 1942. At that time all hospitals operated at 110 percent capacity. The city had a ratio of 1.7 beds per thousand population, compared with a war standard of 4.0 beds. This shortage became particularly acute when the city was faced with a flu epidemic followed by an outbreak of meningitis. No isolation ward was available for victims of such infectious and contagious diseases. Mobile officials were unprepared to deal with the problems that arose during the war years. The city didn't offer adequate services before the war, and it was overwhelmed by the population growth. The city administration did not have the structure for making decisions; no one assumed responsibility or supplied leadership. The mayor finally took action and eventually established the temporary isolation ward (Loftin, 64–68).

Graduate Medical Education

The basic pattern of modern American medical education was well established by 1920, and it continued relatively unchanged for the next forty years (Rothstein, 153). The first two years of medical school were devoted to the basic sciences, and the last two to clinical medicine. The curriculum was later reversed, with the students first entering the hospital wards and then attending outpatient clinics. This change gave them a chance to see more serious cases with well-developed symptoms before working in the outpatient clinics. While the basic curriculum remained the same, the content of courses changed drastically with the expansion of medical knowledge. The same information explosion also increased the courses in specialty areas and the number of class and laboratory hours (Duffy, 267).

Until 1945, all Alabama medical students had to leave the state for their last two years of medical school. A large percentage attended Tulane University School of Medicine in New Orleans, Louisiana. Of the five physicians included in this book, three attended Tulane: doctors Arthur Wood, Ernest G. DeBakey, and Samuel Eichold. Of those, only Dr. Wood was fortunate to attend Tulane during the tenure of both Dr. Rudolph Matas and Dr. Alton Ochsner. These two men were responsible for molding generations of physicians.

Dr. Matas was a world-renowned surgeon. All of his years of practice were spent in New Orleans at Tulane. He was deeply respected by all his students and associates. It is not an extreme statement to say those who knew him well idolized him. He is often referred to as "the father of modern vascular surgery." In New Orleans, however, he was also known as an old-time physician "whose province was the human skin and the contents thereof." Dr. Alton Ochsner succeeded Matas at Tulane. He was on the faculty at the University of Wisconsin when Tulane University offered him the chairmanship of its medical department, the position Dr. Matas was preparing to relinquish. It was a hugely controversial appointment.

When Ochsner arrived in New Orleans in 1927 to take up his position, he was barely past thirty and an unlikely prospect to succeed the idolized Matas. Other more experienced and local surgeons, each with his own following, had hoped to step into Matas' shoes. Ochsner found unfriendly rivals even within his own department. Dr. Arthur Wood, a Mobile native, recalled, "Dr. Ochsner came in and there wasn't a surgeon in New Orleans that would speak to him … He didn't have a friend." However, by 1938 Ochsner had become the most influential practitioner in New Orleans. While Tulane did not have its own hospital at the time, Ochsner succeeded in organizing one of America's premier surgical teaching programs at New Orleans Charity Hospital.

Years before, in Mobile, the state's first medical school had been suspended in 1919 (Jordan, 16). The faculty and students had performed their clinical work at Mobile's City Hospital, also providing that facility with a medical staff. After the medical school closed, it was necessary to replace the college's visiting clinical staff with a regular staff. The City Hospital staff duties were divided among the local physicians, each of whom spent three month long rotations every year providing free coverage to the community.

Much later, in 1939, application for internship at City Hospital was made by three men: doctors Socrates Rumpanos, Woodrow Eddins, and K. J. Compton. During the next year, there were five more rotating second-year interns, each having served at Charity Hospital in New Orleans under Ochsner's instruction (Wiseman, 44). This pattern continued and contributed to the high quality of care offered in the Mobile area. When returning to practice in Mobile after World War II, physicians were responsible for staffing the Marine and City Hospitals. Throughout the years, it continued to be understood that this work was in addition to a physician's regular practice.

While supporting the community hospitals, surgeon Dr. Ernest DeBakey thought it also necessary to support the surrounding rural areas, ultimately exerting a profound influence on health care in southwest Alabama. He and Dr. Vernon Balovich, an anesthesiologist, often traveled to rural towns to perform procedures for those who didn't have access to care. Through that experience, he witnessed the shortage of doctors practicing in rural areas and continuously sought to change that. Later, in 1997, he and his wife established the Ernest G. DeBakey Charitable Foundation to offer education to physicians who serve in the underserved areas of south Alabama.

World War II didn't bring immediate changes to medical education, other than speeding it up. The prerequisite of a bachelor's degree for admission to medical school was reduced in some cases to two years, and the four-year medical curriculum was concentrated into three years of intensive study. The war did bring a renewed interest in medical research, which had a profound impact on medical schools in the immediate succeeding years (Duffy, 267–68).

From 1940 until the closing phases of the Vietnam War, medical education was affected to different degrees by the need for doctors in the military services (Bordley, 399–400). When the Selective Service law was adopted (1940), the AMA insisted on deferments for medical students. Other deferments from military duty were granted to those who were employed in occupations essential to the war effort, such as workers in shipyards, munitions factories, etc. Some deferred physicians came under the heading of those who were providing the only medical service for a community or those who held indispensable positions in medical schools and hospitals. Large numbers of doctors, however, volunteered for military service, and the real problem was to decide how to distribute the limited supply so as to meet both civilian and military needs (Duffy, 304).

When it became obvious that something had to be done to ensure a continuing supply of physicians, the government agreed to grant commissions in the Army or Navy to physically fit students in the junior and senior classes of the medical schools and to postpone their call to active duty until they had completed a one-year internship. Later this arrangement was extended to apply to students in the freshman and sophomore classes.

To provide a continuous flow of students into the medical schools, in 1943 the government instituted a recruitment plan for medical training. Under this plan the Army Specialized Training Program (ASTP) supplied 55 percent of the students for the freshman classes; the Navy V-12 Program, 25 percent; the remaining 20 percent were drawn from the civilian population. The medical schools, many of them already facing financial instability, welcomed this arrangement, since the government not only supplied 80 percent of the students but also paid the educational expenses for those who were selected (Flynn, 321). In 1944 the GI Bill of Rights was passed, providing benefits for armed-services veterans.

During the height of World War II there was a growing movement in Alabama to upgrade medical education opportunities. Governor Chauncey Sparks announced in his 1943 inaugural address that he intended to establish a four-year medical school within the state. By the summer of 1945, the four-year University of Alabama School of Medicine had been established in Birmingham. This school provided the two-year basic science program, originally available in Tuscaloosa, as well as the final two years of medical training that had not existed within the state (Mansfield, 764). If they chose, Alabama medical students were no longer obliged to leave the state for their third and fourth years of medical school.

By the late 1940s, as better-educated interns and residents followed in the path of Rumpanos, Eddins, and Compton and finished their training in Mobile, the City Hospital grew to have approved orthopedic, surgery, and pediatric residency programs. The Mobile community has had a strong interest in medical education long before there ever was a university (Jordan, 18). Graduate medical education was presented in Mobile in spite of the lack of a local formal school due to the concern and efforts of local physicians (Jordan, 25). This type of medical education groundswell was influential enough to generate the necessary community support for the building of a second state medical school, which became a reality in Mobile in 1970 (Wiseman, 47).

Specialization and Certification

The work lives of physicians shifted from general practice to specialization with the development of board certification, and from home- and office-based practice to increasing dependence on hospital privileges. Both shifts are linked to the evolution of organized medicine. The interviews in this book identify the increasing expectations of medicine. At this juncture, older practitioners saw a change in the motivation for becoming a physician, from becoming a physician as a "calling" to perhaps entering the field for status or financial reward.

During the late 1930s, the establishment of specialized fields of medicine and specialty boards led to a fundamental change in the practice of medicine (Little, 321). Specialty boards and certification developed initially out of the need to define and regulate the practice of medicine (Little, 402). A primary cause influencing the development was the growth of specialized knowledge and changes in medical therapeutics, practice, and instrumentation.

Until the turn of the century, when medical knowledge grew relatively slowly, a physician could keep pace with advancing knowledge. Later, practitioners were engaged in an "unprecedented riot of discovery," with rapidly advancing medical and scientific knowledge (*Newsweek*, 42). This coupled with a gradual shift of the location of medical diagnosis and treatment from the home or office to the hospital or outpatient clinic, caused specialization to develop at an increased rate (Little, 318). There was a significant rise in the number of medical specialists, who came into great demand as plans were being made for the return of several hundred thousand battle casualties at the end of World War II (Ginzberg, 522). As instrumentation and techniques developed, physicians required extensive study and practice if they were to become proficient in their use (Rothstein, 72). As the importance of physician education increased, this led to the specialty boards and requirements for continuing medical education. This culminated in a continuous certification process now required of all specialties (Schrock, 785).

As a part of the changes, hospital care became more complex and specialized. As better insights were gained into physiology and as surgical techniques improved, the study of surgery advanced. The evolving treatment of tuberculosis illustrates the developing complexity of internal medicine. In the 1930s surgeons were widely utilizing thoracoplasty in cases of advanced tuberculosis. This operation involved resecting the ribs to allow the lung to contract and rest. In the 1940s the procedure was replaced with pulmonary resection. Later, the advent of antituberculosis drugs after World War II virtually eliminated the need for surgery (Duffy, 257). By the 1950s internal medicine as a specialty had reached a stage where clinical scientists had to limit their attention to certain segments of internal medicine if they were to keep up with new information and improve methods of diagnosis and therapy. Simply stated, they *had* to become specialists (Beeson, 624).

Earlier, in 1915, a National Board of Medical Examiners was established and began giving examinations on a voluntary basis the following year. In the first five years the examinations were taken by only 325 students, of whom 269 passed. As the better schools and state boards recognized the value of the program, more students applied (Duffy, 296). By 1940, the number of candidates taking the National Board examinations had increased to about 1400 a year, or about one-quarter of all medical school graduates. Three-quarters of all American physicians in 1928 had described themselves as being in general practice; by 1942 the percentage had dropped to just below half (Reverby, 181).

Dr. Ernest G. DeBakey, from Lake Charles, Louisiana, graduated Tulane Medical School in 1939 and finished his residency in 1948 after serving in the US Air Force for five years during World War II. There was no doubt that he would take the surgery board exam and earn his certification, even though it was a new development. When he came to practice in Mobile there were very few certified physicians and there was a lot of competition for patients.

But for Dr. Harry Webster and others there was little incentive to become Board certified. "Board certification became a way of detecting two things: it ensured that everybody had a good education that went into it; it also protected the territory from interlopers, which had been people who came in like I did. Just open the door and say here I am, I'm a urologist, don't you forget it. You know? But, that would not have worked . . . for me if I had wanted to go to New Orleans. But it worked for me here because I had. . . established a presence with the community. They knew who I was and what I was and whether I was able to do that."

Initially general practitioners were skeptical of the value of specialization (Rothstein, 72). The economic concern was that specialists would leave general practitioners with nothing to treat. The traditional path had been for a physician to begin practice as a general practitioner, distinguish himself in a field, and then gradually limit his practice to that field (Rothstein, 73). Dr. Webster planned from the outset to become a general practitioner. When he returned to Mobile in 1941, "surgery was done by the general practitioners; obstetrics was done by the general practitioners. There wasn't hardly anybody who had a clear practice, maybe there were two or three . . . That was it: if you were in medicine that was it. Nobody asked me what I wanted to be."

Prior to World War II, many physicians went into practice immediately after receiving their MD degrees. The degree and the successful completion of a board examination were all that was required for licensure in many states, though some states required an internship as well. After the war, very few were willing to start their practice without an internship.

With each passing year more and more went on for residency training in medicine, surgery, or one of the specialties. By the 1950s those who had gone to medical school prior to 1920, when general practice was the common objective, were rapidly dying off or retiring. Communities that had two or three general practitioners in 1940 found themselves without even one generalist 25 years later.

Post–World War II Years

The face of health care continued its change in the era after World War II as nurse's work changed with the status and salaries of nurses increasing. Hospitals added to their housekeeping staffs and no longer expected nurses to scrub and clean, do laundry, and make beds. Registered nurses moved into management and aides and practical nurses handled routine patient care. Following the Depression and World War II, nursing careers were enhanced by hospitals—but the stratification of staffs limited nurses' scope and authority, and that chafed.

The same changes followed physician specialization: many returned from World War II to open offices in downtown Mobile, creating an attractive central location where a larger investment in office equipment further increased specialization. This is where patients began to say they were "going to the doctor's office" and no longer "calling the doctor" for home care. Hospital care and medical specialization developed hand in glove: hospitals offered the facilities and equipment and physician specialists admitted patients to use them.

The individuals in this book started in a profession dominated by general practitioners and returned from World War II to one dominated by specialists. They left Mobile when practices were home-based and returned to work in hospitals and offices. Medical economics shifted from patient payment directly to physicians to inflation of medical costs that coincided with health insurance. Medical interventions ranged from the introduction of antibiotics to a growing range of technology influencing diagnosis, monitoring, and therapy. Hospitalization came to be an expected and an accepted alternative to home care. Health care practitioners came to realize the inflation in patient expectations which meant an increase in their own status and wealth—also meant a distancing in their relationship with patients. The distancing reduced the personal part of medicine which was essentially a belief in healing power, which some said was the greatest weapon against illness. Many felt the exquisite change in patient relationships after insurance became widely available.

Nursing Training and Practice

Closely related to the building and expanding of Mobile's hospitals was the development of nurse training programs and of nursing as a respectable occupation for women. Hospitals' early dependence on the labor of student nurses later shifted toward hospital employment of graduate nurses. Nurses' careers changed from private duty in the first half of the century to work in hospitals and physicians' offices after World War II.

During the 1900s, hospital administrators had realized the value of trained nurses and they knew their nursing schools provided a cheap form of labor (Moiden, 22). The original concept of the nurse training school had been one where classroom and practical instruction would be given. The truth is that most hospitals provided little or no formal teaching and relied largely upon what was essentially an apprenticeship. By providing room and board, hospitals were gaining the services of young women for incredibly long hours per day (Duffy, 281).

Nearly 60 percent of all the hospital beds in the country in the early 1930s were in hospitals with nursing schools; 73 percent of those hospitals had no graduate staff nurses and only 15 percent had four or more. Many hospital officials regarded the idea that they pay for a nursing service as "unreasonable" and saw the student service as an "inalienable right" (Reverby, 188). In the early 1930s, nearly 12 percent of the private-duty nurses surveyed were working 24-hour shifts; in 1932, less than 12-hour duty was almost unheard-of. Many nurses thought a 12-hour shift represented a decline in their service to the patient, or that limiting their hours would mean insufficient work. Fifty-hour weeks continued to be common until after World War II (Reverby, 186–87).

Until the Depression, nurses worked as direct employees of the patient and were called private-duty nurses. During the Depression they began to staff hospitals' nursing services. As the Depression continued, hospitals grew. Patients could not afford the private home care of physicians and nurses and had to seek charitable services in the hospital. The graduate nurse who could not find work as a private-duty nurse had to return to the hospital for a job (Reverby, 180).

During these years, the change from private duty to hospital staffing took place, and it was not easy. Nurses were forced to accept the necessity of a greater division of labor in the hospital workforce: they worked less as overall caregivers and more in specific areas. At the same time, hospitals had to be convinced that graduate nurses, along with other levels of nurse workers, were a cheaper and more dependable, disciplined, and skilled workforce than students (Reverby, 183).

Although educational programs at hospital nursing schools improved, the clinical experiences of most nurses were geared to the service needs of their hospitals. Student nurses rarely received clinical training that was unprofitable to the hospital. Hospitals with large surgical services gave their students a great deal of surgical training; municipal hospitals with many chronic patients emphasized long-term care. In practically all hospitals, students spent as much as 20 percent of their time making bandages, mending rubber gloves, dusting, sweeping, cleaning lavatories, putting away linen, and sterilizing equipment (Rothstein, 138).

During the 1940s, nursing school rules and regulations became more firmly established. Tuition for the training program usually included room and board, uniforms, books, and so much a month for insurance. Students were required to live in a dormitory next to the hospital and had to check in and out. In the second month of school, students were assigned clinical duties. The students and RNs took care of all the patients around the clock, seven days a week. There were no nurse's aides. During the first year of training, students worked in the hospital six and a half days a week. If their afternoon off happened to fall on a day that classes were scheduled, they had to attend class (Roberds, 4).

Margi Gatti, RN, was born "up the street from where the Mobile Infirmary was later built". She became a nurse, training at the Providence Hospital Nursing School in 1943, and grew to manage the operating rooms and teach other nurses at Providence Hospital for 16 years. She entered nursing when student labor staffed a hospital and the physician was king, and when assigned a task she had to fly by the seat of her pants until she completed the job. Reviewing the nursing practices of that time is an exercise in patience for twenty-first-century health professionals:

> When giving an injection of morphine, the student would drop a pill into a reusable glass syringe, connect the parts, and then go to the sink. They'd run the hot tap water, aspirate about a cubic centimeter, and shake the syringe until the pill dissolved in the water. Then, they'd place a sterile cotton ball, moistened with alcohol, around the needle and give the "shot."

> Most surgical patients were admitted the day before the operation. There were no intensive care units or recovery rooms. After surgery patients were brought immediately back to their rooms. They had to stay in bed for a week. On the eighth day, they were allowed to dangle their legs; on the ninth, they could sit in a chair; on the tenth, walk around the room, and by the 11th day, they could stroll in the hall with assistance.

> Twice a day, in the morning and afternoon, IV fluids were administered. Solutions were infused from glass bottles—sometimes up to 1,000 cubic centimeters over about an hour because intravenous therapy was not continuous.

On night duty, when there was spare time, nurse trainees would make small pill trays out of scrap paper. Or they'd clean the used rubber gloves, dusting, repacking, and resterilizing them. If the gloves were torn, they'd cut the tips off and put them aside for use as finger cots (Whorton, 33).

Hospitals did not have to raise wages because they controlled the nursing labor market. Low pay, long hours, split shifts, authoritarian supervision, and rigid rules continued to plague hospital nursing. By 1946, for example, staff nurses were averaging 87 cents an hour, and one in four received less than 75 cents. In contrast, a typist could earn 97 cents or a bookkeeper a dollar and 11 cents, for much less arduous work (Reverby, 192).

Integration of Hospitals

Hospitals in the late nineteenth century were charitable substitutes for homes. They changed in the mid-twentieth century into highly specialized, technology-driven institutions. In Mobile this transformation represented changes in the expectations of health care professionals as well as patients. Mobile's hospitals became a visible sign of its "modern development." The hospitals also represented the established racial structure, which was soon to experience a far-reaching change.

A fight aimed at discriminatory practices in American medicine and health care took place following World War II. The principal targets were the all-white medical society and the rigidly segregated Southern hospital (Beardsley, 2001, 38). While quiet, this fight was as important to blacks as the more obvious and dramatic struggles highlighted in the daily news. It took place in pages of medical journals, at professional meetings, and in talks between physicians and hospital administrators. The falling of the barriers in the South was in no small part due to white physicians themselves. They were human, and as such shared the racist assumptions of their upbringing and communities.

As medical professionals they also recognized the need to set aside racial practices in favor of medically sound practices. Dr. Harry Webster tells of this evolution of personal and professional values. "And so I really felt that it [the Mobile Infirmary] was worth staying lily-white and I tried to keep it that way as long as I could. But there came a time when anybody had to know that there had to be a change, including an old country boy like me raised up there in swamps of Conecuh. Exceptions provided. There was nothing to be ashamed of . . . But it was a change and one that was hard to come by when you have a lifetime of apartheid . . . The law said equal was separate. But of course it never was. It was awful hard to get equality."

In contrast to medical schools, hospitals presented a much more complex problem for integration. It was difficult to change traditional relationships in hospitals that served the entire community (Beardsley, 2001, 42). The hospitals of Mobile served a population of about five hundred thousand, of which one-third was black. Health care in Mobile had always been divided strictly by race. The 540-bed Mobile Infirmary, the dominant institution in the region's social and medical hierarchy, served whites only. The 35-bed Saint Martin de Porres Hospital served private paying blacks of Mobile and was the only facility where black dentists and physicians could admit and treat their patients. Two additional hospitals served both races: Mobile General Hospital, a 247-bed county facility for the indigent, and Providence Hospital, a 262-bed facility operated by the Daughters of Charity of St. Vincent de Paul. Care in these two facilities was strictly segregated by race. If, for example, there was an overflow of black patients in Wing 7 at Providence Hospital, they were supplied with beds in the hall, even though beds lay empty in other, white wings of the hospital (Smith, 154).

Chandler Bramlett, administrator of the Mobile Infirmary, identified his problem with integrating the hospital as one of timing. "We knew . . . that we were going to have to admit black patients. But it was a question of being able to time admission with the acceptance of everybody else. The doctors and the community, too . . . The whole area was going through change, it wasn't just Mobile Infirmary. The whole social chain, everything was being changed. Well, I guess accepting change on anybody's part is difficult at times. It was difficult for the community; it was difficult for the individuals."

Years later, before it was certified to receive Medicare funds, a hospital had to do more than have a plan to end discrimination—it had to demonstrate nondiscrimination (Ball, 63). The four hospitals in Mobile were among the 327 still awaiting Medicare Title VI clearance in 1966. A bitter battle of wills followed during the rest of the year. Later, quietly, without a formal negotiated settlement, the Infirmary was notified of "interim" Medicare certification that would provide Medicare payments to the hospital retroactive to February 1, 1967. The government had retreated and full certification for the Infirmary with Medicare began in July 1967 (*Mobile Press*, 1).

The Integration of Hospital Medical Staff

By the turn of the century, changes in patterns of practice and medical education were set in motion by an attempt to deal with the inadequacies in medical education and patient care. Hospitals became the training grounds for the major teaching programs. Being able to treat patients in a hospital became vital to a physician's professional standing and economic growth.

Following the Flexner Report in 1910, only two medical schools remained to educate the majority of black health professionals. A dozen or so schools in the North admitted one or two black applicants each year, but none of the white medical schools in the South offered that opportunity. Following the four years at medical school, internships and residency positions were even more limited, and staff privileges in anything other than a poorly equipped all-black hospital did not exist for black medical graduates in the South.

There were three patterns of providing hospital services to black patients in the South. The all-black hospital was built exclusively for black patients. The physicians and nurses in many of these hospitals were white; in others they were biracial or black. The mixed-race hospitals were of two types. The predominant type segregated blacks in separate wards, such as all-black wings and basement and attic wards. The other type had separate buildings attached to the main hospital, or separate buildings located on the hospital grounds. Generally only white physicians and nurses were admitted to the professional staffs. In all-white hospitals, predominate in the South, blacks were refused admission in all but the most extreme situations (Reynolds, 885–86).

A black man, Dr. James A. Franklin practiced in Mobile for 50 years. The son of a slave woman, he set up a medical and house-call practice in September 1919. Dr. Franklin's legacy is one of quiet, steadfast strength, committed to providing the best medicine he could in an area where for decades the hardship of race included the inability to be admitted to hospitals. During this time, most blacks needing medical care turned to Dr. Franklin.

The Southern black physician's greatest handicap was his inability to practice in white hospitals. Every institution, public and private, followed the custom of restricting facilities to physicians who were members of local county medical societies, affiliates of the AMA. Since no county organization in the South admitted black members—and they would not do so until after 1950—doors of established hospitals were closed to black practitioners. Even after some white hospitals began admitting black patients into highly segregated wards in about 1930, Negro physicians were still turned away, effectively excluding black physicians in the 17 Southern states (Beardsley, 1986, 79).

Black medical societies were created out of necessity. Black hospitals were also developed out of necessity. By 1910 almost one hundred black hospitals were in existence. While providing better care for patients and facilities for black physicians, these hospitals also contributed to medical education by increasing the number of internships and residencies open to blacks (Duffy, 287).

The World War II era marked the beginning of a new effort by black physicians to gain professional recognition. Whereas only 356 blacks were commissioned as medical officers during World War I, in World War II the figure was around six hundred. While a token number of black nurses were allowed to enlist in World War I, in World War II the figure was around five hundred (Duffy, 287). As a physician member of the Army during World War I, Dr. James Franklin was never called "Doctor" because he was black. His wife, Marguerite Franklin, stated, "They never would recognize him as a doctor, but they made him work on those soldiers as a doctor. But they called him a sergeant during World War I. Yeah, but they would not recognize him. He had a friend from Detroit and they happened to be in the same regiment and both of them were named sergeants, not doctors."

Prior to the 1950s, black doctors in Mobile didn't have access to the city's hospitals, so they treated patients either at home or at infirmaries set up by private physicians. The situation changed in Mobile in 1950 with the opening of St. Martin de Porres Hospital. It wasn't until 1964 that other hospitals in Mobile started opening their doors to black doctors and their patients.

Currently

Mobile's health care history has seen tremendous changes and growth from the sleepy port town of the 1930s. Today the city is a regional center for medical care, research, and education. There are more than 850 physicians and 175 dentists practicing in the area, and most are affiliated with one or more of nine hospitals serving Mobile. In addition, there are many outpatient surgical centers, emergency clinics, home health care services, assisted-living facilities, and nursing homes. Clearly Mobile's history created a generous launching point for today's health care resources. The issues identified here shaped the men and women whose lives are in this book. Their legacy—their decisions and choices—transcend health care evolution, expectations, and expertise. Understanding where they came from and how they assessed these developments may shed light on our understanding of how we got to this juncture in our own crossroads.

CHAPTER 2

Arthur A. Wood, MD (1905–1999)

Surgeon

Springhill College 1924

Tulane University Medical College 1931

Opened Mobile practice 1937

Interviewed over a period of days ending 6/23/94 at 89 years old

I was born right here in Mobile, 1905. My mother and father come from Michigan. My mother was from Kalamazoo and my father was from Hastings, a little town out close to Kalamazoo. My father was born on a horse farm. They had great big draft horses, these big old Clydesdales with hair on their feet. They raised them. Back in those days they didn't think much about education. They were farm people especially. He didn't get but a third-grade education and yet he was one of the smartest men I've ever seen.

He had a blackboard down in the basement when we lived over on Springhill Avenue. He had a blackboard down there and he'd say put up six digits in three columns: six down, three columns. We'll start here and you put down the figures and just line them up. When he got through, he had them added up in his head. I never have learned how he did it. He'd tell me himself that he didn't know how.

When I was taking calculus—trying to figure a problem at home, sitting there, sweating it out. He looked over my shoulders and said I don't know how long it's going to take you to get it, but the answer is so and so. I thought he must be crazy. I struggled about another hour or so and came out with the same answer. He just looked at it. His mind worked just like a calculator. He multiplied everything by tens. And if you wanted to multiply two numbers like 96 and 42 or something like that, see he'd multiply 90 by 40 and then six by two. He could do it in his head, you see.

My father was almost insane on the idea of every male child having to earn a living from the time he could start eating and sleeping. Well anyway, he figured out things for me to do and he had a rule: he wouldn't give you any presents; he wouldn't give you anything, except for birthday and Christmas. The rest of the time you had to work for it. When I was about seven or eight, he said, "You got a horse." See, we lived on Houston Street and the only thing there was behind that on Houston Street all the way to where Murphy High School is now, is this big vacant land, just pasture land. We get out in the pasture and he says I got you a little horse. You see he worshipped horses. One thing he believed was that if you couldn't have a horse, you wouldn't be worth a damn.

He said, now I got something else for you. I said what's that? He said investments. You can invest in a pair of saddlebags. He said you've got a newspaper route with about 125 papers to deliver in the morning. In the morning, I got up and rode that horse. I had to ride to a certain place up on the corner of Dauphin and Houston; the papers would be left. I had to go up and pick up the papers, and I had to roll them and do them like that. Then I'd fly to Newman Street, the horse just sitting on it. He knew after the two or three times he'd done it, he knew it better than I did. We'd have to hit porches on both sides.

Mobile didn't have any paved streets to amount to anything by then. I was living on Springhill Avenue when Mobile Electric Company blew up. Of course we just had one light bulb hanging down in every room. That is the way it was in those days. All the old chandeliers and stuff had been set up for gas. If you had gas pumps running, you could get gas long before you could get electricity. Kids didn't have much fun after school in those days. Most all of them worked. Everybody had something to do. They weren't home. I don't think anybody got out and ran the streets like they do now.

When we got on Springhill, I started down at Barton Academy about then. Anyway, my father told me to sell my horse and I sold him and stopped my paper route. I rode a little bicycle down there. You couldn't take a horse down there to go to high school. I had to buy the bicycle. All the things I got, I went from one investment to another. My dad was basically a salesman. He owned Wood Printing Company. He didn't know a damn thing about printing. He had a business partner that knew all about the printing business. His business partner got tuberculosis and died and Pop just kept the business and ran it. He got to where he could do almost everything in there. I ran everything in the print shop, except the cutting machine. He told me you're not going to get your hands around that cutting machine. It cuts paper that thick. Anyway, he let me run everything but that.

But, he said what you need to do out here on Springhill Avenue; we've got a lot of room out here. Some of these people got cows and he said you don't have a cow. You ought to go in the dairy business. And I said oh Lord. He picked out a little Jersey cow. She was just like a pet, just like a dog would be. She just loved me and followed me around. Anyway, Josie—we named her Josie—when she was fresh she gave four gallons of milk a day. And I milked her at 6:00 in the morning and at 2:00 in the afternoon every day and afternoon. If I was a half hour late at 2:00 in the afternoon, Mama told him about it and he'd give me hell for that. Cow's already gonna get you in trouble and you're gonna have a sick cow with a damn stiff udder and all that stuff. I really could milk that cow. I'd get out there and clean her up at 6:00 in the morning and sit a stool up under her and let her chew on some food. I milked her all the way through high school and Springhill College. Milking that damn cow.

When I went to Tulane finally and I caught the train, I said I'm not ever going to make another garden. I'm not every going to keep another lawn.

I'm not ever going ride another horse that's living in the stables. I'm not ever gonna milk another damn cow. And then when my wife got sick with Alzheimer's disease, I found myself doing everything but milking the cow!

I was at Springhill College from 1922. I just took premed. Two years. I went to Tulane and worked in between. I did everything on God's green earth to earn enough to get through Tulane. I was going to pay for my own education. My father told me, he told me if you get in trouble, I'll lend you some money, but I'm not going to give you anything. I paid for my education out at Springhill myself. Yeah, with that cow.

Why was I a doctor? Well, when I was 11 years old, my eleventh birthday, the old man says you're getting to be a pretty good boy now, what do you think you're going to be when you grow up? I said I'm going to be a doctor. He said a doctor? You don't know anything about doctoring. Why do you want to be a doctor? I said I don't know. I think that's what I want to be. He said, the only time you ever had a doctor was when you broke your arm and they put you to sleep with some chloroform and tied your arm up when you was five years old. I said I know it but that's what I want to do. I never had wanted to do anything [else] since.

I had to stay out of Tulane for two years. I didn't finish the schooling until 1931. I was supposed to finish it in '29. I ran out of money. Things were going poorly. Things were bad. That was the Depression. My father had promised that he would carry me through my junior year. He got interested in oil leases here in Mobile County and he bought leases all over the place where oil was found 20 years later. But they didn't drill but two thousand feet, then they drilled twenty-one thousand feet 20 years later. Anyway, he lost everything he had. He went broke. And he didn't tell me he was broke. I was writing checks and he was supposed to be putting some money in the bank. The next thing I knew I had checks out. I was trying to find what was wrong and I called him and asked him what was wrong and he said he just didn't have the money. Couldn't get it. So I had to stay out of Tulane for two years.

To make money I built the Merchant's Bank Building almost by myself! They had a fellow by the name of Moore that came down here from Virginia and he advertised in the paper for somebody to run this motor trench pump. It was a huge motor, electrical motor, that took 440 volts of electricity to run it and it would pump three thousand gallons of water a minute. I read the advertisement and went down there to see about it. He put me on.

As soon as I quit the job, I went over to New Orleans to see the dean of Tulane Medical School and I said well I'm ready to come back. He said, you studied any better? He said you'll have to teach your junior year. I said I don't have time to do any of that. I'm going in and I'm sitting in class. He said you can't do it. I said I think I can. He said how are you going to do it? I said, if you let me I'll stay over here in New Orleans through the summer and go on up and take all my junior class examinations over. I took them all in September. I took them all over again and got better grades than I did the first [time].

Dr. Ochsner came to Tulane when I was a junior. He was only 32 years old. Dr. Rudolf Matas had been head of the surgery department at Tulane for 60 years. He was one of the finest surgeons and one of the most brilliant men in the whole world. He was just known all over the world. He spoke seven or eight languages and read two or three more. He just had a brilliant mind. One time when I was a junior student, there was three of us together, we happened to get on a ward in Charity Hospital the same time he was making rounds.

He was by himself and he had a nurse with him, but that was all, not even an intern or anybody. They came up on a bed, blanket on him, this comatose patient on it, just dying, in horrible shape, didn't know what was going on or anything. All over him was his own fecal material and everything, he smelled bad, and he looked bad. It was just a horrible sight. We had this one young fellow in our class and he had more money than either one of the other two of us together.

But anyway, he kind of stood back and so Dr. Matas looked at him and said, "Examine the patient." He was just horrified. He couldn't stand the idea of putting his hands on that horrible mess and Dr. Matas said, "Son, there but for the grace of God lies you." I said to Dr. Matas, can't we wash him off a little bit first. He said, yeah, I think that's a good idea. He called a nurse over and we washed the patient down.

This is a man that was really a great man. He turned New Orleans into the best medical center in the United States and Tulane was the best medical center. He was chief of surgical services at Tulane for 32 years and stayed pretty well in charge for another 25 or 30. It gives you the whole story of medicine for the twentieth century. He loved this medical school. See he's the one that trained all the surgeons in New Orleans. And then he called up Albert Ochsner in Chicago and said, "Who can I get to be chief of surgery for Tulane?"

Every doctor and every surgeon in New Orleans thought he was going to be the chief of surgery, because Dr. Matas trained them all. He went up to Dr. Albert Ochsner in Chicago and said, "Albert"—they were good friends—"I want you to pick you a young man to take over my surgery department." He said why don't you take my nephew, he's in Switzerland now. He's about finished up over there, why don't you take him? And Dr. Matas took him over all his own people. They thought he was crazy. They thought he had gone nuts. And that's when Dr. Ochsner came. So, of course, you just don't find it, all those men Matas trained: he loved them, they just loved him, too. But they were just flabbergasted.

Dr. Ochsner came in and there wasn't a surgeon in New Orleans that would speak to him. They wouldn't have anything to do with Dr. Ochsner; nobody would have anything to do with him, even the residents and interns and everybody else. He didn't have a friend. Mims Gage came and Dr. Ochsner took him on. Claude Wright, who was my roommate, and I were on Dr. Ochsner's ward. Now we never had examined a patient, starting our junior year. When he walked in there—the first time we'd ever seen him—he said, for each patient in this ward I want you to have them all worked up by tomorrow and I don't want you to look at a chart. We had to do our own laboratory work. We had to do work-ups for 18 patients and we worked back there all day and all night

Dr. Matas, he's the one that said to the three of us young junior medical students, "There but by the grace of God lies you." That's all the teaching I got from him. And every time I got mad with a patient, which really wasn't very often, I would remember Dr. Matas' words. I got mad with a lot [of] people, including patients!

I had a time with my preacher. The preacher, Dr. Seever, was my Baptist preacher. One night I had this smart-alecky 19-year-old boy that thought he was a big shot. He had a fight with his girl and he'd taken some iodine and smeared it around on his lips and mouth and made his mother believe he'd committed suicide. Made his girl believe that too. See, anyway, they brought him into Mobile Infirmary. I was over there taking care of another emergency and they asked me if I'd take care of this kid. I started out by saying, what'd you do? He said, I did what I said I'd do. And I said, you swallowed some iodine? He said, yeah. I said, how much did you swallow? He said, oh, big bottle full. I said now I'm gonna wash your stomach out. He said you and who else? I said me and the crank off this table if necessary. I wanted to crack him upside the head. I couldn't stand him, a smart-aleck kid.

About that time, his mother came in. She was a cute little old grandma with her hair all up in curlers and a floozy-looking thing over it, the funniest-looking thing you ever seen. She come in crying over her boy trying to commit suicide. He started laughing at his mother. Boy that's when I really got mad. I'd already washed his stomach out. And I said you damn little no-count, too bad she didn't miscarry you. And I looked over and the preacher was standing there in the room listening to me. I said well preacher, I guess you heard some pretty unministerial language and he said yes, I certainly did. I said, you don't like it? He said, I don't like it. I said well that's kind of the way I am. Nobody laughs at their mother. I've been taught better than that.

Anyway, about two or three weeks went by and the preacher came into my office and sat down and said you know that boy that you cussed out that night, he cried for three days after that when you told him, it was too bad that your mother didn't miscarry you. I said, I meant it. Anyway, he said, you know what he's done? He's joined the Marine Corps and he says he hopes it'll make a man out of him. I said, well what do you think about that? He said, well all I can say is, you do it your way and I'll do it mine.

When I was in medical school, we decided—there was 18 of us, 18 of us students in the same '29 class—decided we were going to go to church every Sunday, a different church every Sunday. We went to eleven different churches. We went to every kind of church there was. We tried to get in a synagogue. We had a Jewish boy. We went to all of them. We came to the unanimous decision that all of them thought that they were the right way to get you to heaven, number one. And number two, they all needed money bad. That was a pretty good part of my education. All at once, I realized that there were so many ways to get to heaven. So many much easier ways to go to hell.

Ochsner was a wonderful fellow. He had an ugly temper. He'd give you hell. He'd tear you to pieces, sometimes not justified. They had an amphitheater: you put all the junior and senior students in there in kind of a clinical pathological conference. You'd go out in the hall and you'd have a patient out there for you and you'd had about 15 minutes to make a diagnosis on that patient, do the best you could, see. And you couldn't look at his chart. So, there was a student in there, a junior student, who had his patient, the patient was deaf and dumb and he didn't speak. Dr. Ochsner thought he had him, see. And when he came in he had the history and the physical almost perfect. And Dr. Ochsner just threw a fit. He said, you cheated; you had to look at his chart. You couldn't have known that much about him, he's deaf and dumb. About that time, the patient started doing this hand stuff and then the student started doing it back to him. Ochsner said, "I beg your pardon, I'm sorry."

Dr. Ochsner, when I went back for my senior year, he was always friendly with me and all that but he never was like he was before. Never quite forgave me for leaving. See I wouldn't ask for help. I think if I'd asked for help, somebody would have financed me. Damn pride. I've given up all kind of things because of pride. When I graduated from Tulane, there wasn't any member of my family there, nobody there. The girl that I'd been in love [with], we broke up long before. Anyway, I sat there. The auditorium was so damn hot. It was terrible. When I finally got my diploma, it occurred to me everybody else [was] being hugged and kissed and carrying on. I walked across the street and sat in the park and wept.

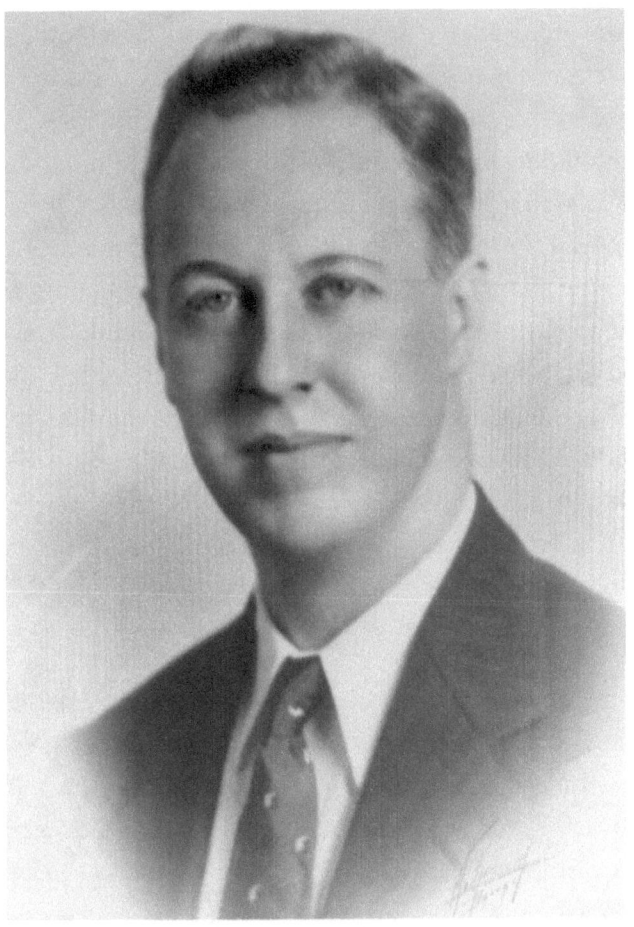

Dr. Arthur A. Wood graduating Tulane Medical School (1931)

I came back to Mobile in '31. I had my internship here at the City Hospital. I had a residency lined up at Touro Infirmary in New Orleans with Mims Gage. My father was having dizzy spells, real bad dizzy spells, and they lasted for a long time. They were having a hard time treating them for him and there wasn't any symptoms of this other thing. I mean he had a little trouble with his heart at that time, too. So I decided to come home to be with him, instead of taking a residency at Touro. I came over here and took it at City Hospital, internship. I made 40 dollars a month as an intern. Forty dollars a month.

Well, the second day I think it was of my internship, they had a man working at the filling station across the street from City Hospital. Someone threw a tire tool down on the cement and it skidded across the whole place and hit him in the back of the ankle and cut his Achilles tendon and they brought him on into the hospital. Well, I checked him out and it hadn't been completely divided, it was a fresh wound. I cleaned it up, washed it all up, put Novocain in there, fixed his tendon, and put a cast on it. The next morning Dr. Hannon came in and said what happened here? I said his Achilles tendon, he said who did it? I said I did. He said, "You did it? Oh, my God, you just got here the day before!" I said I thought I knew how. He told me, you'd better damn sure know. Anyway, the third day came around, I said Dr. Hannon, I'll take a look at this wound and see how it's doing. He said no I'd like to see it myself. It was slick as a button; see, it healed up. Back about two or three years ago, I ran into this old black boy. He said Dr. Wood do you remember me? I said no I don't guess I do. He said, I'm the fellow you fixed that afternoon. I learned that from Dr. Ochsner.

The Conniff brothers were the ambulance drivers. They were characters, Bob and George. Talk about having experiences. George was the nice one, Bob was kind of rough. George, you'd think he was a bastard, but he'd been a marine in World War I and he was just as nice as could be. He carried a .44 pistol automatic; carried it a long time in the ambulance in a holster in case he got into some real bad trouble. Because every now and then you'd get somebody wild or something. Anyway, George kept talking about all his experiences in World War I, how many nice German soldiers he killed and all that kind of stuff. We got a call down on Government Street between Royal and the riverfront to an old three-story house down there and it was an emergency call. George was driving—he drove nights and Bob drove in the daytime. So he drove down there and he got that gun out. He said, I don't like the looks of this place. I think there is something wrong about this. Maybe somebody's trying to get some dope over here or something. We don't know what it is. He said, I'm gonna carry this gun. So he went up these three flights of steps and he had that gun in his hand. There was this bunch of trash up there. They wanted some dope. And he pulled that gun and aimed it at them and he said now I'm gonna tell you something. I killed some good men in Germany and I'll kill the whole G-damn bunch of you. I said, no you won't, for God's sake let's back out!

Have you heard about Edna Greenough? Edna Greenough ran a whorehouse: Edna Greenough's whorehouse. She was on the corner of Canal and Warren Street. Anyway, it was about 11:00, 12:00 at night, we got a call. I was on the emergency service and it was Edna Greenough and said it was a real emergency could we please come quick! So George was driving the ambulance and we got there and this great big black woman stood in the front door. She was proud to see us and waving us in. She waved us in and had a house full of furniture and red carpet up the steps. I went up there and came to the door. There was this great big poster bed in there with a man on it buck naked, deader than a doorknob. Standing in the corner was this little old 17- or 18-year-old girl. She didn't know what was going on. She was scared to death. Anyway, Edna come in there with us and I examined the man, listened to his heart and all that, asked how long he'd been dead, there wasn't any sense in trying to revive him. That's when I finally looked at his face and he was one of my father's best friends.

I motioned to George that he was dead. Told him to take the little old girl out and wrap something around her. She was scared. George, when he got back to the room, I said, where is his car? She said it's in the alley back behind the trees. It's the only car in there. I said can we get up and down the back steps? She said, yeah, I think so. So George went down to get the ambulance livery, but he couldn't carry it up the steps. So I said anyway we've got to get him dressed. You never had a time until you start dressing a man from socks to vest and all and tie.

We got everything on him and we took him and walked him down the steps. That's what we did. We got him out to the car and opened the door of the passenger side and we put him in the car and set him in there. I got the car and Bob pulled up behind the alley and waited until I got out and I took him out just around the corner from where his car was. They were good friends of mine. Anyway, we got about a block from where I was going to stop, I started slowing down. Bob was about two blocks behind me. Anyway the sirens came screaming up and we opened the door and took the body out and put it on the livery and put it in the ambulance and took him to the City Hospital. We left his car where it was.

We got to City Hospital. I called his daughter and I told her that we had got a call from somebody in the neighborhood; somebody ran in and said it looked like somebody was terribly sick in that car. And that we'd gone out there and it was her father. She fainted. So, his son was about five or six years younger than I was, I called him and told him the same story over again. And anyway, a month or two later, I guess it was, Edna came through the hospital. She said, I'll never forget what happened that night; that she owed me something, that she wanted to do something for me. And I said, I don't think there's anything. I thought she was gonna offer me the services of her house. She didn't go that far.

She said well, I'm gonna come talk to you. I said all right. So she came in later and she said you know prostitution may be legal. She said the legality of it is built around the fact that we have to have our girls examined regularly. She said, I want to bring my girls to you and you examine them. It was the height of the Depression; I was seeing everybody and everything that I could. I said, I'll help. Bring them in and I'll check them for gonorrhea, check them for syphilis and whatever. And so this went on for about four or five months I guess. I charged them ten dollars apiece cause they were doing well, it was helping out. The next thing I knew Edna had told that story to someone and he spread it all over the town. About five years later, I was still getting business. My wife came to downtown to shop and we went over to Morrison's to eat. I was walking to the automobile and one of those little girls went prancing along by and she said hello Dr. Wood and I said, hello, honey, how are you doing? She said, I'm fine. Frances said, "Who is that?" and I said oh a professional acquaintance. She said, "Your profession or hers?!"

When I started practicing I got an office in the Van Antwerp Building. I didn't have any money. Instead of a waiting room, they stood right in front of the elevator on the fourth floor. Herman Kurley, the dentist, had the office to the left as you go out the elevator and I had the one to the right, one room. I had that one room divided into an examining room and a little cubbyhole office and a little old tiny lab room. I had all the stuff I needed in there, see. I hired Agnes Renthroe as our receptionist. We didn't have a nurse; we couldn't afford one. I just let Agnes come in while I was examining patients and all that just to have a female with the patient.

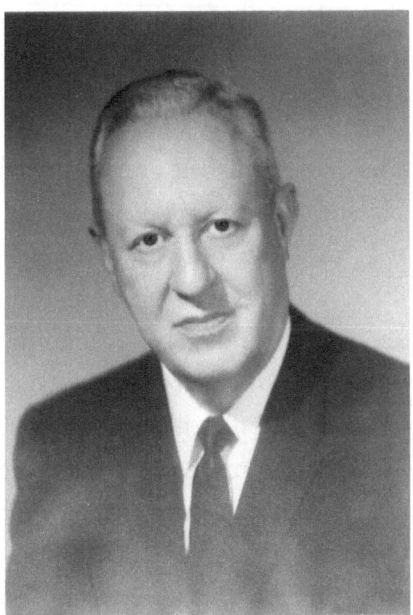

Dr. Arthur Wood during the 1940s (date unknown)

Kurley decided that he was going to get gas anesthesia to pull teeth. He told me, I'll leave this office open and if you ever need this gas machine, I'm telling you to come over and get it and use it. So, it was a Saturday afternoon, a really nasty day and nobody was in the office except me. Agnes was off and I was going to spend some time reading for Sunday. Anyway, in walks this dirty little old boy about 12 years old and he's crying. He stuck up his finger like that and it's swelled about twice as big. There's a big old rag on that end and he was crying and he said this finger hurts me. I need something done for it.

I said, why don't you go to the City Hospital? He said, they just told me to soak it in Epsom salts. I said, where do you live? He said, I don't live nowhere. I said, what's your name? Where's your mother and father? He said, I don't have any. I said, what do you do? He said, I sell papers. I go to the *Press-Register* and I sleep on the rags down at the *Press-Register* pressroom and they take care of me. Sometimes they feed me a little, give me a little breakfast. He was young, you see. I said well this thing is infected. You can't do anything with local anesthesia if the patient has a bad infection. I said, you ought to be put to sleep. He said, I'm good, get it out of here. You wouldn't dare do this today.

I got that gas machine and pulled it over to my office and put him up on my examining table and put him to sleep and split that thumb wide open and got a little old pussy junk out of it and stitched it up and dressed it. He stayed there a little while, waked up good and I saw him every day for two or three weeks, except Sunday. No penicillin, no sulfur, no nothing in those days, see. You had to get it well. It took about two months I guess to get well. Of course, he didn't have anything. I didn't charge him. The man from the *Register* wrote me a letter thanking me for what I had done. Anyway, he got well. I guess it was maybe six months or close to a year later. I got to getting all kinds of patients, a lot of children and people on the ships came in from down at the State Docks. We saw a lot of people from down at the State Docks who paid cash.

We had a ship captain in there off of a French boat. I said, who the hell sent you? He was from down at the State Docks. He said there is a dirty nasty little orphan boy down there who sticks his thumb up in your face every time he sells a paper and tells what you did for him. The captain said if he's good enough for him, he's good enough for us. Call that advertising. You don't ever know who's going to be there.

I did not charge the blacks over one dollar for anything done for them. Most of the blacks, I did for nothing. They couldn't afford anything. I never turned down a patient in my life on account of money. I never turned down one in my life. But I did not charge them anything. I had them by the hundreds, charity cases. All my life, I had a percentage rate of charity cases of over 40 percent of my patients. Two people and I shared a surgical service at City Hospital, see, and I spent three months a year working for that hospital, City Hospital, day and night on the surgical unit, for free. All of the doctors did it at that time.

It was fun before the Medicaid and the insurances came in; when you would do something for charity. What we would do, for a charity patient: on Sunday morning, I would do it routinely, I'd call my nurse, my anesthetist Ms. Rice, and say, "Ms. Rice do you want to do something for Jesus today?" And she knew what I did. Providence had already asked me to take the case. The Sisters at Providence would always call me for their charity patients.

Sister Kraswansky: I loved her more than anyone else. She was there when I started practicing at Providence. She ran the Providence Hospital. She was about 69 or 70 years, a big fat motherly Irish woman. Just a wonderful person. Anyway, I came into Providence, because John Wilson called me when I was finishing at City Hospital and wanted to know if I wanted to help him in surgery. John Wilson and H. G. Coleman were the only two trained surgeons in Mobile, all the rest of them were general practitioners that liked to call themselves surgeons. Some of them were pretty damn good. But anyway, I came over to Providence to help John Wilson. I worked with John Wilson for five years. He taught me a whole lot. I took care of all of his patients; I'd go to visit them, do physicals.

Christmas came, I didn't have anything. Ten dollars was like a thousand almost, it was just unbelievable, so poor. I was in the Van Antwerp Building for five years before I paid the first month's rent. Jim Van Antwerp used to come down and apologize to me because I couldn't pay him. He'd tell me, say doctor, you got a huge practice, it's gonna pay off. I said, that's what I hope. Anyway it was Christmas, she had her head down between her hands and she was crying. I said, what's wrong? A patient had just given me a one-hundred-dollar bill. That was a whole lot of money and I had the one-hundred-dollar bill just squashed down in my pocket. I said, "What's the matter with you?" and she said, I got all these patients that we need to feed and we don't have any money. We're just like you, we don't have any money. I said, I've got some money. She said, "you have?"

She said, I don't want your money. I said, I'm gonna tell you something, Sister: I'll get it back in the next 24 hours. She said, you're kidding. She said, let me know about it. I went down to the office. Lying on my desk was a great big box with five hundred dollars' worth of surgical instruments that a doctor in Lucedale had sent me for operating on his wife. We had to have our own instruments. I picked up the phone and I said, "Sister, I got it five to one."

Then, we got in the habit, she called me and said, "Dr. Wood do you want to do something for Jesus?" and I said, I do my best work for him. She said, we got this patient that hasn't got anything and we wondered if you would operate on him. I said yeah, I'll do it. This went on all through these years. This is one of the reasons why I stayed with Providence. I knew how sorry things were a lot of times.

Providence Hospital and I were just one thing through all those years. They had one sister one time, in all those years, that got to me. I guess it was about three months or something like that and I went into her and I said, "Do you want to do something for Jesus?" This is what we always said. She said, "What are you talking about?" and I said, I've got a thyroid patient that had hyperthyroidism and I've got her all worked up and ready, the anesthesia is gonna be for nothing, the surgical assistance is gonna be for nothing, I'm gonna be for nothing, are you gonna take her for nothing? She said no, you do too much charity in this hospital. I said, I don't know what you're talking about, Sister. She said, you've had six patients in this dad gum hospital in the last couple of months that have been charity patients and I said, I don't know who you are talking about. So I didn't pay any attention to her. I told A. J. Brown about it; he got all upset. So he checked all this out. He came to me and said you know who these six patients were? I said no. He said Sisters of Charity. St. Louis. He said, let's go see her. He walked in there and told her who the charity patients were. He said, "Now Sister, do you want our patients or not?" She said, well of course I want them. He said, then you take our charity.

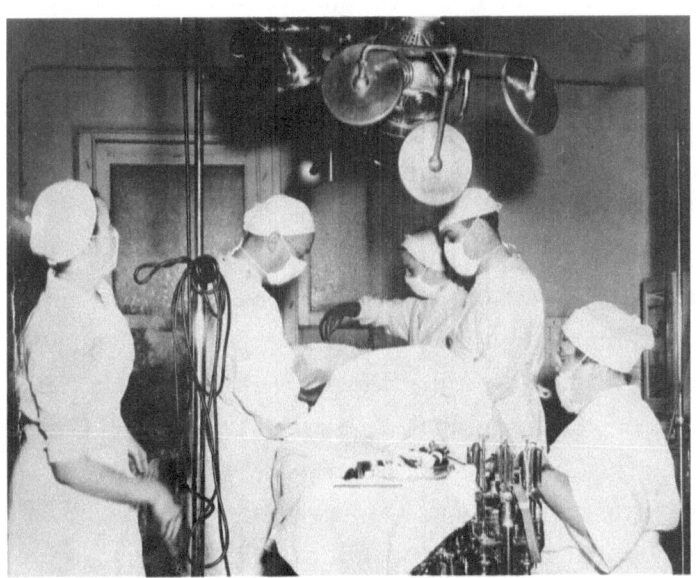

An operating room at Providence Hospital (left to right): M. Gatti, RN,
Dr. Brown, R. Wood, RN, Dr. Arthur Wood, and nurse anesthetist Vera Rice,
CRNA (date unknown)

Politics doesn't start in the hospital. Politics start in society. When I came here, there was a doctor by the name of Dr. J. D. Purdue. He was rich. His brother, his older brother, didn't even practice medicine. He was a doctor but he didn't even practice medicine, he was just making money. But anyway, he let J. D. run the show. But J. D. was a real politic. He brought men into Mobile and encouraged them to practice certain forms of medicine, who were not specialists but they called themselves specialists. J. D. verified them as specialists.

By doing that, he gave the general practitioners a chance in things they never had otherwise. One guy for instance was supposed to be a urologist. He never looked through a cystoscope in his life. He was a clap doctor. That's all he was. He was a nice guy, a real pleasant person and a pretty good practitioner. J. D. got him to be classified in everybody's mind. Another guy came in, he wasn't anything but an obstetrician. Dr. Robertson trained him for surgery. Charlie Robertson was a trained gynecologist and so this guy never did get to where he could teach. He got to where he could lay the instruments on a hysterectomy, but he couldn't do a vaginal hysterectomy. J. D. had a group, Avrill and Segrest. Segrest was a trained internist, but he had him in his group. All these people voted like J. D. wanted them to vote. There was six or eight of them. They ruled all the politics in the medical society for years. He decided who'd be on the Board of Surgery, he decided who'd be president of the Society. Everything. Anyway, it went on all the time before the war. Nobody paid much attention to it because there wasn't much you could do. I broke with him one time before I went to war. He called me and said, Dr. Wood you are going to have a hard time. I said, I'm sorry that's just the way it is. After the war, I came back. I never got over it: he took one of the little contracts that I had away from me. He talked the company into taking it away and giving it to another doctor.

Anyway, so I came back from the war.

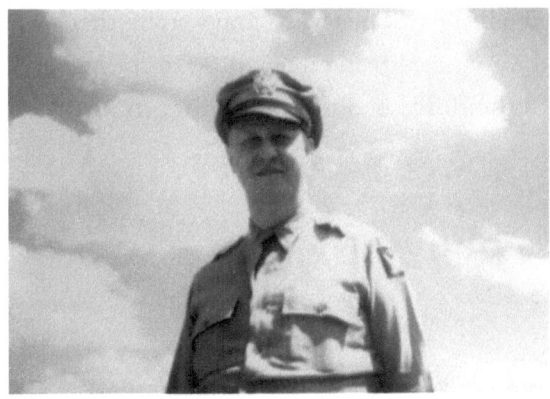

*Dr. Arthur A Wood, Air Force lieutenant colonel, taken while
at Roswell Army Base in New Mexico (1943)*

The Medical Society was pretty upset. Joe Little said everybody that sits on the Board of Surgery has been there for more than 20 years. He said we've got to cut off Dr. Carpenter. He was a sweet little old man, he's been on it for over 20 years and it's time that he's off, too. This year, we want you to run against him. I said, why do I want to run against Dr. Carpenter? He said because you're so damn mean. And I said, I don't know whether I want to be that mean. I like Dr. Carpenter. I don't want to hurt him. And he said, we want to stop this thing of J. D. telling who's gonna be everything. So they ran me for the Board of Surgery. I won by one point. I got on the Board of Surgery. At the first meeting I told them, I said I'll tell you what my purpose is: the Medical Society thinks all you folks have been serving too long on this board. I said I'm going to try to make a motion immediately that each member of this board go along because it is the right thing: nobody on this board will serve more than two terms of three years. Boy, they knocked me down. They knocked my teeth out.

A couple of physicians were very excited when I said this. They thought the board had done very well and they wanted to keep it like it was, which was very shortsighted. I got up and I asked if it was proper, could I make a minority. I made a minority to support the new Society and so that's just what happened to all them. They had a gravy train, that's what it amounted to—control of the Society. I made the motion to the Society that they abide by my motion to the Board of Surgery and they did. And we won.

CHAPTER 3

Marguerite Wiggins Russell Franklin (1906–2005)

Wife of Dr. James A. Franklin, Sr.

Emerson Institute 1924

Pratt University in Brooklyn, New York 1926

Married Dr. Franklin 1951

Interviewed 4/19/2000 at 95 years old

Dr. James Alexander Franklin, Sr. (1886–1972)

Lincoln University, Philadelphia 1911

Michigan University Medical School 1915

Began medical practice in Mobile September 1921

I'm Marguerite Wiggins Franklin. I was born on Old Shell Road between Springhill and Florida Avenue. 1906, September 3. I'm 94 years old. I'll be 95, September 3. My daddy was 95 when he had a heart attack. Of course, my mother, she died earlier. She fell on a banana peel getting on the streetcar. She hurt her stomach and it formed into cancer. Somebody had gotten off the streetcar and dropped a banana peel and she went running to get on the streetcar and she fell. And she always suffered with that side. She died when she was around 65.

I finished Dunbar School first. Then they had a school here at that time named Emerson Normal Industrial Institute and the American Missionaries was over that school. They seemed to be Episcopalian; maybe they were Congregationalist. We first had that school on Government and Ann Street—it was called the old Blue College. It was on Ann right across from Weineker's Delchamps. Mr. Caldwell who was later principal of Emerson School finished there, Ms. Josephine Allen finished there, and Dr. Wilkerson finished there. Finally, they burned it down. Then they moved to Scott Street. They burned that one down, but the missionaries didn't stop. They continued on to building the school back and we had school in churches until that school was finished.

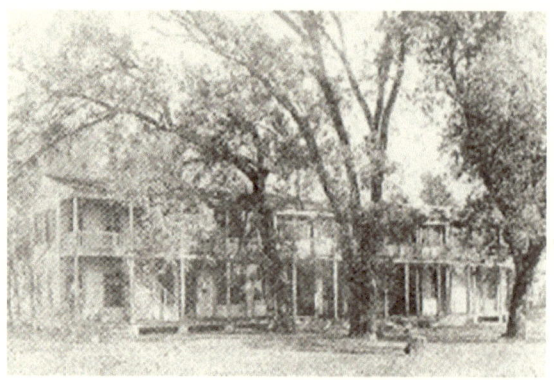

Emerson Institute High School, located later on Scott Street in Mobile, Alabama

We had all white teachers. Then in the late years, we had about three black teachers, Ms. Singleton, Ms. Kingsley, and Ms. Patton, Dave Patton's wife. At this school they taught you, they had a trade you could take and the regular academic classes. And cooking and sewing. So I took the trades, cooking and sewing and my academic work and pedagogy to prepare you for teaching. And after you finish, you could teach anywhere in Alabama and not take a test. My daddy wanted me to continue on, so he was determined, at that time it was Tuskegee for blacks. But my instructors, this cooking teacher was Ms. Singleton, she was black; my pedagogy teacher and my sewing teacher were white. They said that I would be going backward if he sent me there. They wanted me to go to their school, which was Pratt University in Brooklyn, New York.

Papa said no, not my baby. She's never been away from home. And they pleaded with him and made him understand. They said now Mr. Wiggins, you've got the means and she wants to go—why don't you send her? So he finally made up in his mind. I went to Pratt in Brooklyn, New York in 1924! I was 18 years old. Oh, it was something. But I got used to it and I went on. It was big to me. Of course, I was from Mobile. At that time, it wasn't Mobile, it was Crichton, Alabama.

My father was first a dairyman on Dauphin Street. He came here from Monroeville, Alabama. He worked for some Catholic people and they saw he was very smart. Dr. Wiggins's daughter taught him to the fourth grade. That was as far as she could teach him. After he would do his chores, he'd come in and she saw he caught on things just like that. She saw he was a great mathematician. He taught me before I went to school. I could count and almost read the paper. He was a very smart man, just gifted, that's what he was, gifted.

So Father McLaughlin came there to see them—because he would get milk for the Sisters. They rode around in a buggy at that time and would go to a different place to pick up milk. So, she called Papa in and told the father, "He's so smart," says, "I just don't understand how he catches on so easy." So, he said, I could use him at Springhill College. I think he can get a better job up there. And he did. Do you know what he did? He let him sit in the back when they were giving brick lying and cement finishing classes and he listened and learned. He couldn't go to school, but Father McLaughlin told him, you be back here like you are working—and listen. And he had a photographic mind. He remembered everything that they did up there. So they started building on campus and they put him out there and they said that if you let him see the building and give him the measurement of that building, he could tell you how many bricks.

When I met Doctor I was living in Chicago because I was separated from Dr. Russell. I was working at Kellerman's, one of the largest stores there for dressmaking and dresses and furs and things like that. I had seen Dr. Williams's daughter; she invited me to come play bridge. So I did. Then I met Doctor; his wife had died. So he was my partner.

I was here in Mobile, visiting. Arial Holloway, she invited me to this party and I met him. He said, I remember you when you were 16 years old. I said, no, I don't remember you. He said I certainly remember you because you had a touch of pneumonia at Dunbar High School. I did. I was going to school one morning and I fell out in the hall and they sent me—he was living right here, but in a smaller house. He said, I waited on you right here in this house, 355 North Ann Street, when you were 16. He said you're just the right age of the wife I want because I don't need any more children. I was 45 at that time, when I married him. So I said, I certainly don't remember that. Then, it came to me. I surely did remember because I remember I had on my sister's stockings. We wore stockings back then that had laced all up. I was in the senior class; I thought I was grown then. But I had put a hole in the toe there. I told the teacher don't take my shoes off. She said why? I said because I've got a hole in my stocking and that doctor will see it. But you know I had forgotten all about that he had waited on me. Sure enough he did, when I was 16 years old.

I lived in Chicago for five years and then I came back and married him. We courted for just a few months. We married in August. I could go by the clock: at nine o'clock every night until I married him he telephoned. He was so afraid I was going to change my mind! And at nine o'clock when the phone rang, I said, "I know." He called me on the phone until I came back and married him. Come to find out, he was one of my brother's best friends. I didn't know that. He said, I know your family. I know Willie well, said we ran around together. I was in Chicago and I didn't know anything about that. He was a wonderful man.

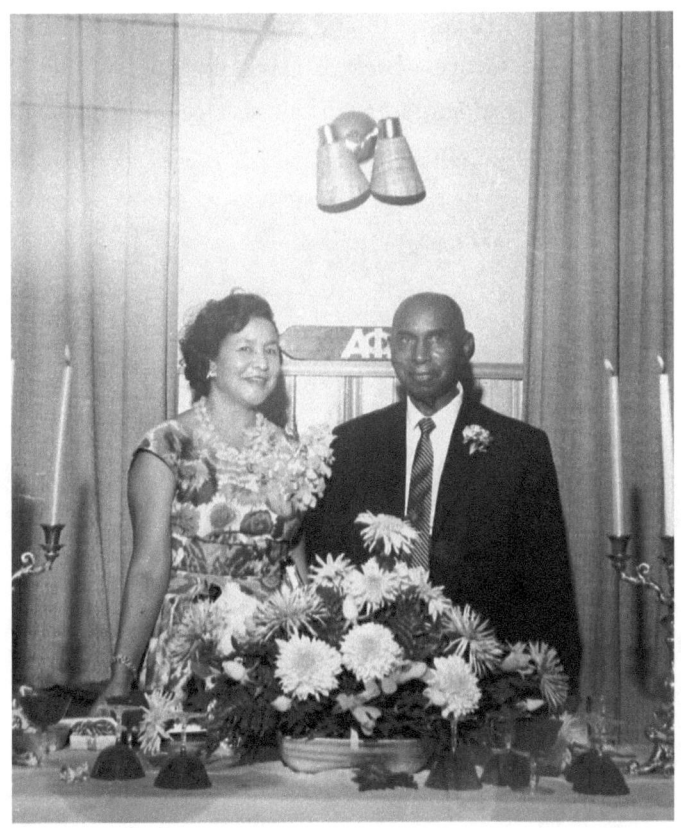

Dr. and Mrs. James A. Franklin (1951)

He loved people. He charged three dollars per patient from the beginning until he died. He never charged these poor people any more to go to their house. And he went to their house because I drove him in the last years. He got kind of feeble and he wasn't able to drive. He was so feeble that I would take his bag and put it on the porch and somebody would come out and get it. He just loved people. If they had the money, it was all right. If they didn't have it, it was all right with him. He said people in Mobile made me what I am today and I want to give something back to them. That's why we let his office, right there on Davis Avenue and Cleveland Street; built him an office up here, so he wouldn't have to go upstairs. He opened that office up for doctors to come in and treat patients that didn't have any money. The Sisters of Martin des Porres asked if it was all right for the doctors to come in and help the people over on the north side, over there in the Grove—back of Davis Avenue. We let the people come over and different doctors gave their service and that's the way the Franklin Memorial Center started.

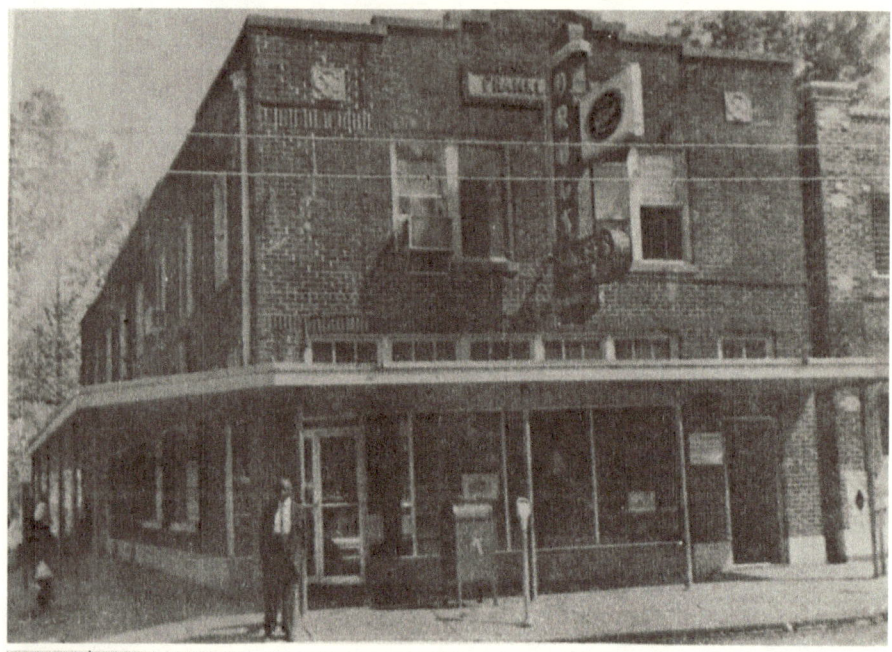

THE FRÁNKLIN BUILDING ON DAVIS AVENUE AND CLEVELAND STREET--This building was heavily damaged by fire, especially the ground floor businesses. The up-stairs compartments were mostly smoke damaged which included: A doctor's office, Dr. J.A. Franklin; a certified public accountant's office, Thomas Reed and the Non Partisan Voter's League, John LeFlore and others. The above building has been sold to the Urban Renewal for about five weeks, according to the former building's owner, Dr. J.A. Franklin. The large sign on front of the building says: DRUGS- FINLEY'S # 3 and behind it says THE FRANKLIN BLDG. The 81 year old physician can be seen standing by street marker near left end of picture at corner. (Staff photo by E. Madison Cockrell)

Franklin Building on Davis and Cleveland (date unknown) Dr. James A. Franklin practiced medicine in Mobile for 50 years. He set up a medical and house-call practice in September 1919. Dr. Franklin's legacy is one of quiet, steadfast strength, committed to providing the best medicine he could.

When he took sick, he knew, but I didn't know, that he was as sick as he was. He had heart trouble. He never told me nor his children. I knew it was something wrong with his heart. He finally told me, I want to make my will. He called his son from Kansas and his daughter and the two

Dr. Goodes, he worked with them up in his building. He called them. He made his will about three months before he died. He signed it and everything. He said, "Now listen, if anything happens to me, I don't want you to go through my books and collect any money that these people owe me." He said, "When I'm dead, my bills are paid. People have paid me everything they need to pay me." And I didn't. And many a one owed him.

He was born in Tennessee, Chattanooga. He left there after they put him in the Army. They wouldn't call him a doctor in the Army. They never would recognize him as a doctor, but they made him work on those soldiers as a doctor. But they called him a sergeant during World War I. Yeah, but they would not recognize him. He had a friend from Detroit and they happened to be in the same regiment and both of them were named sergeants, not doctors. After he got out—he came home and burned his suit! He said they wouldn't recognize me and made me do the work. He said it's unfair. So he burned his suit. I never did see it, nor anyone else. He was with his other wife at that time. When he died, they sent a stone and that had "sergeant." His children said, "No. We'll buy our own stone for our daddy, because he was a real doctor." They called him sergeant. That's the way he was done in the Army.

He went to Lincoln, to Swift Memorial College, and finished junior college there. His mother wasn't able to send him to college and I think it was the Episcopalians that sent him on to college, sent him clothes and things. I heard a friend of his, who went to college with him, Reverend Williams from Tuscaloosa, said how hungry they were at times. Said they would go out in the field and eat raw corn they were so hungry. They didn't have enough food for the children at Swift in Tennessee. So he left there and he worked all the summer and he made his way to Lincoln University in Philadelphia. He was a straight-A student. Those people at the Episcopalian school they sent him clothes and paid for his books and things and he stayed in school there.

Then when he came home, after he finished there, he went home and his mother asked him what was he gonna do and he said, I guess I'll have to stop and work. I would like to go on to be a doctor. He said, I think I'll go to Mehary. She said no you'll be going backwards if you go to Mehary. Because Mehary wasn't up to par at that time. That was before World War I. So, he talked to the professor there at Lincoln University and he got him registered at Michigan University and that's where he finished up, a straight-A student. Because I went to the 50th anniversary and one doctor was living that taught him in 1914.

He told me that Doctor was the smartest student that he had ever had at Michigan University. He said, I taught him from the beginning until the end. He said he helped these boys, one fellow was a cripple. Some mornings he'd get up, he couldn't go to school. They were all white; he was the only black student in that class to finish. This fellow, when we went to the 50th anniversary, the class of 1965. That's when they had their 50th anniversary. They said we are honoring Dr. J. A. Franklin this morning because our instructor told us (This man was still there at Michigan teaching! He couldn't hardly walk!), he said that he told us that he is the only man that stood up in class and named every bone in the body. That's why he's the only student he has ever given a straight A to. I told his children, you all don't know how smart of a daddy you have. He's a smart man, because I heard it myself, from Michigan University. And he was so humble. Nothing like that fazed him. I was so proud of him.

Doctor came to Plateau after he waited on a white woman in Evergreen, Alabama. That's where he was staying when he came back from the Army. He was living in Evergreen when he left the Army. They needed a doctor there. He was there practicing. All the white doctors had given this lady up. Said they couldn't do anything for her. She had pneumonia. There was no cure for pneumonia back then. This man, a rich man, up there north of Evergreen, and he was in the kitchen one morning so burdened down, said I'm going to lose my wife—gave her up. And his cook said, you may not want him, but I've got a good doctor. He said, who is it? She said, he cured my little boy of pneumonia. He said, I'll give him anything he wants if he will come see my wife. Doctor knew what he was getting into; they slipped him in there at night.

So he waited on her. And somehow it got out and the Ks got behind it and ran him out and this man got him out on the train. He said he doesn't know why, but he just got off when the man said Plateau. He had heard somehow Plateau being an African town. So he said he got up and got off there. He said he was walking down the street and this little girl saw him coming and told her father (Mr. Shamburger), "Daddy here comes a man all dressed and got a bag in his hand. He looks important to me!" And he said her father came out on the porch and he made himself acquainted with him. Doctor asked him where he could find a room to stay. This man in Evergreen had given him some money, gave him quite a bit of money. He wanted to find a place to stay and he said, "I'm Dr. Franklin," and he made himself acquainted with him. He said well you can stay here with us until you find a place. He said it just looked like the Lord was opening a way for him.

I got a picture of him in the office. He made an examining table out of an old dining room table in this little hut out there in Plateau. Oh, it was so funny when he took me out there and showed me everything where he started. He walked from Plateau to Mobile, and was known for curing people. He cured that lady of pneumonia. After his name got out in Mobile, the people here in Mobile started calling him, wanting him to come in to see them. Mr. Shamburger had a job and he couldn't bring him in his buggy every day. So he walked from to Plateau to Mobile nearly every day waiting on people. That's a long way.

Then he finally bought him a horse and buggy. Then he sent for his wife and children. I think he said he had four children born in Evergreen. He had sent them to Tennessee, because his wife was from Tennessee. He sent them on to her parents to live there until he could find a place here in Mobile. So he sent for them to come on down and they did. But anyway he stayed out there and then he decided that he had so many patients in Mobile, he decided to come in and he took that money and bought a Chickasaw house and had it moved here on 355 North Ann Street. He stayed in that house until he started making enough money. This house is built around that Chickasaw house. That's the way he moved here on Ann

Street and built this house. The last five children were born here in this house, the midwives. Doctors didn't deliver children back then.

You know Dr. Russell was over [at] the Carnival Association. You remember reading about him? He just died about four years ago. At the end, I had to take care of him. He didn't have but one child, my daughter, and she was a counselor in the public schools in Philadelphia and there wasn't nobody here to look out for him. She said mother I can't leave my job because it's almost time for me to retire. She's 65 years old herself. I had my niece go over there and see about him when his other wife died and there wasn't a soul out there but him. People criticized me and said, I just don't see how you could do it. I said, I'm a Christian. What he did to me, he's got to suffer for that. I said my daughter cannot leave her job and come down here. Somebody's got to look out for him. That was my daughter's father. I couldn't turn my back on him no matter what he did to me. I had forgotten about that, because I was married to a good man.

I worked with Dora, the first Mrs. Franklin, at the YWCA. I'm a charter member of the YWCA. We were on the YMCA board. Mrs. Mitchell, whose home is on Springhill Avenue, gave the Negroes a house on St. Francis Street. Well, gave us a building, the black women, a building on St. Francis Street, and I worked with her. She was the secretary at the YWCA at that time.

Then they moved out on Somerville. I got my gold pin, YWCA. Cooper and I worked and raised money for the YMCA on Dearborn Street. Worked right along with him. We raised seventy thousand dollars, the two of us. It was when they opened that new place on Dearborn and Congress in the sixties. Gary helped good. We worked right along together. He put me over all the ministers and the teachers. And they pledged three hundred dollars apiece. And all of us, we pledged one thousand dollars: Cooper and myself and several others. We pledged one thousand dollars. We raised that money and we got that building because we had to—because the city would give us so much if we raised so much. And we were determined to raise that money, so we really went out there for it. Built a branch out here on Dearborn. That's where the Negroes used to go. Everything was segregated. Everything in Mobile was segregated. That's the way it was.

A lot of people, the doctors would help these people. There were so few Negro doctors back then but they did everything they could to help the people and tell them how to live. I know my husband, Doctor, came home one evening and said a lady had died. He said, do you know what she died from? Collard greens. He said she didn't cook them long enough. He would tell the people even how long to cook collard greens: for three hours because they have live spores in them, and he said cook them three hours. He said, don't you ever cook collard greens unless you cook them a long time. A lot of people here in Mobile from the Indians they found out how to use herbs and things like that. They took better care of themselves by doing that. Because if they had to wait on the doctors to come to see them and do for them, they wouldn't.

Before Martin des Porres black people had a separate—my husband had a patient at the Providence Hospital. And he sent her out there and they couldn't take her in the hospital, but they put her in a back place they had. And when Father Warren came along, and he told Father Warren—Father Warren was over Most Pure Heart of Mary School on Davis Avenue—that this patient really needed care and that he had nowhere to put her and that child was going to die. So Father Warren started thinking about a hospital for Negroes and that's the way we got Martin des Porres (1946). Doctor started it. It's a shame that we can't even put patients in the hospital where they belong. And if they sent them down here at the General Hospital, they were left just laying in the back there. Got a little care I guess, whatever the nurses could do. Only white nurses.

It was pitiful back then. Only God took care of the people. These colored doctors who were able to go to see them: Dr. Williams and my husband, and Dr. Wilkerson and Dr. Brown (he was on St. Francis Street) and Dr. Harris. Those were about the only doctors we had. They just did what they could for the people. General Hospital was separated. Negroes was put in back. Now, my mother, you can see her picture there, now she got better care because she was white.

She fell in love with Papa when they were children. He worked for Dr. Wiggins, that's where we got that name, Wiggins. Dr. Wiggins was in Monroeville and we got the name of Wiggins from him. And her father was Dr. Hawkins, a white doctor in Monroeville. Her mother was half Indian and half white. As a little boy, they would make him look out for Momma because she was a pretty little baby girl. And she fell in love with my daddy.

When they grew up, she was 16 and I think he was, I don't know how old he was exactly. They ran away to Pensacola to marry. When she got to Pensacola and went in to ask for a marriage license, they asked him, this is what he told me: "Nigger, what are you doing with this white woman?" She was quick on the draw, she says, "I'm a mulatta. I'm not white, I'm a mulatta." He says, "I don't believe it." So Papa told him, if you don't believe it you call Dr. Wiggins in Monroeville, Alabama. Cause Dr. Wiggins reared Papa. He really liked Papa. He called him and he said you got a man down here that we're gonna string up. He's here with a white woman. She says she's a mulatta, but we don't believe it. He says, "What's the name?" and he says, "Jake Williams." "Oh, yes, she is. Yes she is. She is a mulatta." And they had the rope there to hang him. He told us that. So they let him go and told him said, "You get out of Pensacola as fast as you can and don't you come back."

Yeah, he got the license because Dr. Wiggins said she was a mulatta. They kicked him right out of Pensacola and he never could go back. He was afraid to go back to Monroeville, so he stopped in Evergreen. But do you know? Her father loved her. It was a hard life for them. Pretty hard, she said at first, with our people and with his people. Because she was really white. Just had that little drop of Indian blood in her. Her brother was the best-looking man I ever saw. I saw his picture. They stayed in touch. I never did meet my grandfather. I was the eighth child. She had nine and I was the eighth. And I'm the only one living. My sister died, 101 years old, about five months ago in Chicago. Her husband was 104, died last month. Yeah, he didn't marry anymore. He loved her and she loved him. He had seven daughters and two boys. All of them are dead but me.

I did a lot of integrating. I integrated with Bishop Smith who was the bishop of Mobile at that time and John L. LeFlore and Gary and I and several others of us. We started integrating and LeFlore would call me and tell me to go different places. He said you're the only one that's got the nerve enough to go and help integrate. I was the first person to go to Van Antwerp Building. Yes ma'am. You couldn't go in there and set up there at the counter and eat anything. You could go and buy medicine or something in the drugstore, but you couldn't sit at that counter. So I had a black Baptist preacher with me and he said Mrs. Franklin, please don't order anything that will take you a long time to eat. They might do something to us. I didn't say a word. So, he went in and he ordered a cup of coffee. I ordered a salad. I never seen a man perspire so in all my life! Perspiration was running off that man and I was . . . But LeFlore told me, he said wherever you go I'm always near or a cop is near you. Said, just holler.

One morning he called me and told me to go to the L&N, this was five o'clock in the morning. They are opening up the railroad station for Negroes. He said Mrs. Franklin please go and get somebody, not your color. I was lighter then. He said get somebody darker to go with you. So I thought about my pastor's wife and I knew she would be in for that. So I called Mrs. Baker and she said yes, I'll go with you, Marguerite, and I said all right then, I'll pick you up in the next hour. Doctor said, where are you going? And I told him. He said I'll just stay here and pray they aren't going to do something to you. He said Lord; I hope you don't get in trouble.

I got up and dressed and went on down there. We went in the L&N station, Mrs. Baker and I. There was four white men in there at six o'clock in the morning. We sat down at the corner and she said, what will you have? I said some coffee. They said, what are you doing serving these niggers in here? She said well I got to. She says they came down last night and said we had to serve blacks. She didn't say black then, she said nigger. Uh-huh. So, two of them said I'll never sit here and drink coffee with "n," you know, "n's," and she said well I'm sorry, but that's my job and I have to do it. The others two fellows sat there and drank their coffee and we drank ours. That's the way we opened up the L&N station down there.

We were the first when we got ready to go to the Medical Auxiliary. Dr. Taylor's wife and Dr. Dickson and his wife, we all went down there. Doctor and I, I said you come on we're going in here because it's integrated. We've got to break the rules and go on in. Let them know that they've got to serve us. So we went on in. His oldest daughter was with us. She said, y'all can go in there if you want to, but I'm not going in there because I ain't gonna let these people shoot me. So I went on in and sat down, then Doctor came on in.

We were going to the National Medical Association meeting. We were going on the train. So we went in there and sat down. The rest of them wouldn't come in there. I tried my best to make them come in there. They wouldn't come. They didn't do anything. We all sat there together. We got our tickets and everything and when we got ready to get on the train, we got on the train. We integrated them that day. Yes sir, I integrated the Saenger Theatre. You know we had to go upstairs. I went on in there and sat down. I never had any trouble but one time. I went out to the mall. The first mall was over on this side, over there where Gayfers was, Springdale Mall. So I went out there and Albright and Wood Drugstore was here then. So I went in there and I had Dr. Battles's daughter. He was a doctor, but he left Mobile and went to Seneca, Alabama, to practice. I had his daughter because she was here going to school with her grandmother. She was one of these little fiery persons. She said I want to be in on it, I want to go.

So I took her with me and we sat at the Albright and Wood counter and ordered a Coke and we were sitting there drinking it. I saw this white fellow looking at me and she was kind of light too. When I got up and left, he got up. Something told me that he was going to do something. So I went on and got in my car. Doctor had given me a big Cadillac. So I got in my car and he was over on the other side of the mall and he watched when I pulled off. I was still watching him in my mirror. He pulled off right behind me. And I went on. I got on Airport Boulevard to come back to Mobile and every time I'd get to a light he would bump me.

So the second light I stopped at, he did the same thing. And she said, ooh Ms. Marguerite, he's after us! Do you think he's gonna hurt us? I said don't worry, I'm gonna get away from him. So I came on down and turned at Sage Street. He kept following me. Came to Ann Street. Now I said, now listen: when we get to Ann Street, whether the red light or what's on, if I see a clear way I'm going on through. Because he's after me and I'm not going by home because I don't want him to know where I live.

So I came on to Ann Street. Sure enough the red light was on. I turned on that red light, came onto Springhill Avenue, and by that time he was coming behind me. There was a red light. I went straight on. I said Lord don't let the cops stop me. I came on through that red light and turned into St. Stephens Road and left and he stopped with the red light. He didn't know where I had gone.

So I went around, she lived back here on Cedar Avenue. So I took her home and I stayed there a while. I told her grandmother, Leanna, I said I'm not going home right away. I'm going to stay here because I know he is trying to find me and she said thank God you all didn't get hurt. He wanted to find out where you lived. I said I know he did, but when he stopped at that red light, I said, I speeded up and went all kind of streets. I don't know how I got here! He looked mean. That's the only trouble that I had.

I was married to Dr. Russell during World War II. A man across the street was working down at the shipyards and he came home one day; he walked all the way home. He said they are fighting on that water down there and turning ships over and barges over. Because we had a lot of Mississippians in here and they didn't want the Negroes to be working on those barges.

You see Mobile was different and apart from the rest of Alabama. We were under the French people. I don't know. We lived together: every neighborhood nearly had white and Negroes in it. We didn't know too much about segregation as these other places like Mississippi did. Out on Old Shell Road, white was on this end and on the other end was Springhill where the whites lived and we just lived together. They'd come to my mother and would borrow sugar. Because daddy kept us, he was a cement finisher and bricklayer, and he was gone all the time because he put that building, whatever you call that, around—in Bay St. Louis—that cement wall. My daddy was with that and he was gone all the time but he left us with plenty of food and everything. We could buy our food by the barrels: barrel of sugar, barrel of flour, and he killed his own hogs and had a smokehouse in the back. He had the man at Springhill College to bring us bananas off of the wharf. I don't like bananas today. I ate so many bananas when I was little. They would come over and say Ms. Wiggins I need a piece of meat for my vegetables, Ms. Tanner and them. We all lived together. Did you know the Tanners out there? My brother and them used to play with them, and they'd play with him. We didn't know too much about segregation like some of those people.

Then they started turning those barges over that those Negroes worked on, but those Negroes were turning theirs over. You don't know how many people died down there in that bay. Very few people know about that. They never published it. No, Langham and them broke it up. I think it was a week. But they broke it up. Some of them Mississippi Negroes left and some of them they stayed here. But Down the Bay, well that was really integrated. But when this integration started where Negroes could move anywhere they wanted, they all moved and moved out. Some of them still live down there. They moved out because the KKKs were after them. You know.

I remember when I was going to school at Emerson . . . in the teens, I went down to Emerson and Papa let this little fellow bring me back because he couldn't take me. We were coming back from a school play because I was in the play at Emerson School. When we got to Shiloh Baptist Church, we saw all of these people coming, dressed in white, coming down from Springhill, coming down Old Shell Road. I told him, that looks like the KKK. We hid up under the Shiloh Baptist Church. It was a tall wood building. It's different now, it's a brick building. We went up under that church and hid. Momma was standing on the porch and she said Lord my child is out there, please don't let them hurt my child. We were up under that church until they passed by. Papa said one of them hollered, "Hey, Jake," because Papa came to the door to see what was going on. He said he recognized that man's voice and he was marching. They had been up and burned a cross on Old Shell Road at a white woman's house because she was a prostitute. Those white women were prostitutes and they were up there on Old Shell Road and they meant for them to move out of that neighborhood.

The KKKs were right here in Mobile. Yes, they were. They were still here. Some of them are still still here! Yeah, because my son came home before my husband died. He said I saw something today that I never thought I'd see. Said a KKK was out there collecting money at the first light after we left the airport. Yes, he said, I never thought I'd see that in Mobile. I said it's here son, it's quiet, but it's here.

Even when LeFlore was living—because this house was the center of every Negro artist that came to Mobile. They stayed here because they wouldn't let them in hotels. We kept Marian Anderson, Thurgood Marshall. We had Jackie Robertson and his whole baseball team stayed here. Football team from California, they stayed here. We had Sugar Ray Robinson's wife. She came to speak for the AKA [Alpha Kappa Alpha], she stayed here. Everybody that came. President Kennedy's secretary stayed here.

We had a white lawyer that stayed here. They told him about it and we came home from playing bridge one night. Doctor liked bridge, I did too. We came home about twelve o'clock one night and I saw a car out there with a whole lot of white crosses. And the man across the street worked for a florist. I said I never saw him bring his crosses like that. I wonder what he's gonna do with so many crosses. Doctor said hurry on and get in the house. He knew what he was, but I didn't. And it was the KKK, because I'd had that white man stay here in this house, that lawyer. He was with Walter White from the NAACP. Walter White, you know, he was just like my mother: he was black and white. He spoke here. And they were going to burn that cross. Doctor came in and put lights everywhere. He put on all the lights everywhere. I came in and said, what's the matter with you? He said Marguerite those are the KKKs out there. So they didn't burn the cross in front of my house. They went around to LeFlore's house. He lived back of me. They burned the cross in front of his house.

They didn't burn the cross in my front yard because they knew that that white man stayed in this house—they thought Walter White was white. They say that he said he was a Negro but he wasn't. He was a mulatto. He really was a mulatto. And he stayed here. So they burned it in front of his house. So after they burned the cross there, LeFlore called Father Foley out at Springhill College and told him they were on their way out there because he was working with the Negroes. They knew he was, Father Foley. Sure enough Father Foley got those students together and they hid behind the hedges and when they got out and put the cross down those boys jumped out and beat the devil out of them. They sure did. They got in that truck and left that cross and never did come back.

We did the best we could. We did the best we could. I think what we did really helped because we integrated Mobile. All those Alabama towns, up to Birmingham and Selma, said Mobile was different than any other city, because we really did integrate here. It was successful, surely did. I think we did a good job and I was right in there with them! My husband, I gave him a lot of trouble. He worried about me, but he didn't bother me. He let me go on and do what I wanted to do. He just knew that I was determined. He found out that I was a determined person and he just trusted me that I knew what I was doing. And so he let me do anything I wanted to do.

We've been through something, but we came out of it. I'm just happy that I lived through all of it.

CHAPTER 4

James Brodie Foster, "Red" (1907–1995)

Fireman in 1932

Part-time ambulance driver for City Hospital in 1935

Interviewed 5/20/94 at 87 years old

I've got to be specific, you know and very careful. What questions I'll answer is truth and facts as I know and not debatable. Yes ma'am, because you know you're talking about way up, the big leagues: the doctors. Whew!

I was born in Tampa, Florida. I can explain why. My daddy, my father, was employed on a dredge boat; dredge Herndon owned by Writtenhouse and Moore in Mobile. And they had a dredge that went down like that [hand movements], operated by a operator on a barge on what they called a scow. And that bucket would go down like that and close it and bring up mud. Digging the channel in places and bring it up and empty it in what they called a scow. The tugboat would take that scow out wherever the authorities told them they could unload it from the bottom. They would unwind cranks to open it in the bottom. All that mud and slush soft coming right out, would empty out wherever they were told to. Had permission to unload that in the channel, Mobile Bay or wherever they were designated to empty that.

My daddy was a carpenter and he traveled on this dredge boat. The name of it was dredge Herndon and Writtenhouse and Moore were the contractors and had a contract in Tampa Bay to do some dredging. And naturally poppa, and my mother, she went out there with him. I think they were married in 1865 or '64. Well, anyhow, they were married.

Poppa's name was James C. Foster. He was a native of Nashville, Tennessee. My mother's name was Amelia Brodie. That's my middle name and my daughter's first name, Brodie Marie, to keep the name of Brodie in the family much as I could. My first daughter was named Barbara Anne. An older lady was superintendent of nurses in the old City Hospital, she named my daughter. That's where my children were born; all three of them born at City Hospital: Barbara Anne and Brodie and my son, James. My oldest and youngest are deceased.

I know it well as I know my own. See, I'm 87 years old. A lot of things I can register in my memory right quick when I hear it. I know it. This lady, it was her and another one. It was ran by and operated by the Sisters of Charity, the old City Hospital. Which the building still remains, but it's changed now to something to do with the state: the Public Health Department. They had St. Vincent's—white hoods like that—nuns. Sister Virginia was in charge when I was a fill-in ambulance driver. The regular drivers were George and Bob Conniff.

They started out at the ambulance service over there which was operated, bought by, and owned by the city. City and county both was in charge of the City Hospital, that's what they named it. That's how they operated: the Sisters of Charity was in authority and ran it. Sister Virginia was the head sister when I was filling in for either one of the Conniffs or Bill Holcombe. He took over. Bob Conniff resigned and went to work with Higgins Mortuary. That's when they were on Government and Washington Avenue.

I was in the fire department. For 48 years, in the fire department. I got promoted while in the fire department. I joined in '32, 1932, and took my pension in '79. That's how many years I was employed in the fire department. And then I was promoted on a civil service examination for a fire inspector and I came out on top on that. And then I was a fire inspector and investigator, too. The origin of the fire, whether it was accidentally; try to determine if possible the starting of it, whether it was negligent, accidental, or purposely, or this that or what, for insurance. It's just according to the nature, the starting of it. You've got to be very careful when you interrogate people and then witnesses, too. Cause a lot of them was death caused by fire and other injuries by fire, the damage by the fire.

The biggest fire? In 1919, June the 21st. Yes, ma'am. Twelve square blocks, lined up.

Yeah, I was 12 years old. My pictures was taken, the back of me and I was standing up looking at the results: the debris, the chimneys, the trees, and what was maimed by this fire. And it began June the 21st, 1919. It started at Cunningham's Grocery Store and Meat Market combination on Hamilton and Madison, on the northeast corner. He was burning; you know in those days they had the kerosene indoors for lights. Yes ma'am, in the square tank.

You'd go get kerosene was the main thing for lamps and so on and so forth to use. Naturally, it'd drip. We had shavings in the store, sawdust, cause it was a combination of meat market and grocery store. So, on this particular day, at 3 p.m. that evening, there's a northwest wind blowing. Well, Mr. Cunningham went out, the fellow that ran the store, and to burn, sweeping up old sawdust shaving and all, and some of it was results of that kerosene tank being inside instead of outside and it was a wood floor. It got paper and all. It was just a grocery and meat market combination, small grocery store, not a large one. Corner grocery we called them in the olden days.

Now, if you're interested in it I can, won't take me long—cause I'm telling you the facts, the results of that fire by experts who investigated it. In those days I wasn't in the fire department then, I was only 12 years old. I was a delivery boy for National Drug Store for Marson Wilkerson, them days they named it, on Washington Avenue. Now. Dr. Wilson ran this drug store. He says, Foster? I said, yes sir, Doctor? I rode the bicycle three dollars a week, after school hours. I was attending Mercer School at the time, Broad and Augusta. He said put the bicycle up, he said Mobile is burning up. Look at it.

We looked and all at it and I remember this: black smoke. Some others in the neighborhood too, they all ran over and got close as we could. Started at three fifteen it burned out by five o'clock. That wind caught it, that northwest wind and the fire trucks, two of them, number three and number five, they were on Franklin Street, about four blocks from the scene. When they arrived—they had horses in them days, you know, horse-driven—and most of the fire department personnel was out at the Monroe Park at the baseball game that evening. Because they could get in on their uniforms.

Some of them, they didn't have radios or nothing in those days. Just had telephones. They called in for help, help, help. Help, quick as they could find out. You could, in case of an emergency, there was a rule in the City of Mobile for the police and the fire department and law enforcement. You could call a taxi to go to the scene when you were needed in case of an emergency. But my golly, by the time you get telephone conversation, here, there, there, not half of the personnel of the firemen were there, but quite a few of them. But they needed everybody for to help cause that fire started at three fifteen and by five o'clock it was smoldering. Twelve square blocks!

By golly, people would get their furniture out on the sidewalk and between the honest people that knew what to do—pick it up. But they had to do it and do it like that [finger snap], you know, to get it away. The northwest wind was, buddy, it was "walking the dog" as we call it. So a lot of looting was going on. Oh, you better believe it. I knew a family that got burned out. They got their phonograph, in those days, you wind 'em up and played records. Held in a cabinet. Whatever else they could get out of the house. Everybody went like that. It was closing in on them, they had to run and leave it! The looting going on. People would take things at all fires, large fires, you could expect that. They found a phonograph down at the foot of Eslavia Street. June 21, 1919. Oh that area was very thickly populated. We took care of some good friends that worked at Hammel's or

Gayfers or at Kresse's or worked somewhere downtown. Two ladies and one of the children was going to school and we lived up on Wilkerson Avenue, right off of Texas Street. Old-time friends and we bunked up together to keep them until things got straightened out.

In 1932, I lived close to the Central Station, that's right there by Ryan's Park. Creighton Towers was a hospital them days, for nervous people, Inge Bondurant, they called them, where Creighton Towers is now, by St. Joseph's Church. I am a member of St. Joseph's Church. I went to St. Joseph's School. And where Ryan's Park is now right—across the street from Creighton Towers is Ryan's Park. Father Ryan's statue: I saw them when they mounted that thing. I was a kid, sticking my nose into this, into that, and all, curiosity. I was one of the ones that happened to be present.

The Central Fire Station they called it, that's the chief's office, assistant chief, and number 17, number five, number three. That's three fire companies in that building. And then the fire prevention office where it is now wasn't on then. That's what's in the Central Station now. But it was a middle market—the big market was downtown back at City Hall. That was the big market. It was vegetables this that and all, rabbits would hang up where you could buy them. Just go to the market, similar to the French Market in New Orleans. Give you an idea of what it was. However, they built the fire station there; named it Central Fire Station on the whole block. That's what it is now. I joined the department in 1932. I resigned and took my pension in '79.

I went regular in the fire department and they'd send me over there to the ambulance when one of the Conniff brothers wanted a vacation or get off or something like that. They would send me over there as a supernumerary driver. On the ambulance. That's how I come to get associated with that operation.

That was in, wait now, went regular in 1935 and I joined the department as an extra man, supernumerary they called it. They had 17 on that board waiting for somebody to die, quit, or get knocked off, or discharged or suspended. Would in their place, extra man, supernumerary they called them. I was the 17th man. I joined '32, went regular in '35. Company number seven. Dan Sermon, former fire chief, he was lieutenant. In those days they had lieutenants and then captains, double shift. He was one of the lieutenants. Captain Brown was captain, Dan Sermon was the lieutenant. One of the boys got in trouble and I was the first on the board to go anywhere regular.

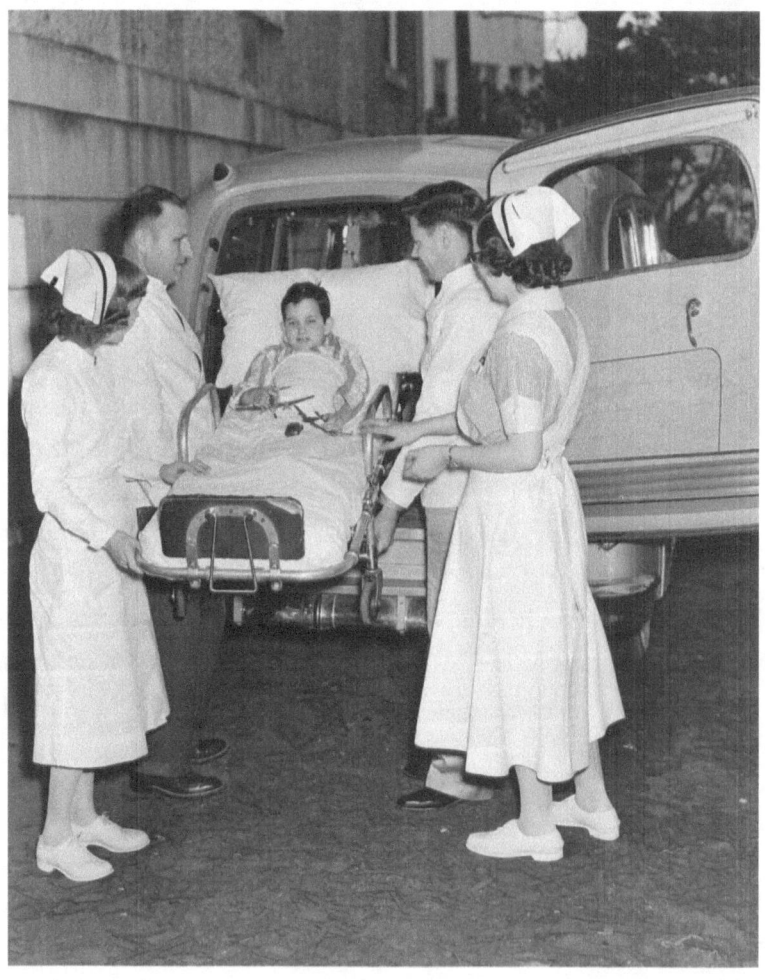

Ambulance at Mobile City Hospital (photo undated). In 1932, Mr. James B. "Red" Foster was a part-time ambulance driver for Mobile City Hospital. His story is included because of his knowledge of the City Hospital and his awareness of the practice and results of home remedies was firsthand.

Yep. Well. I drove the ambulance. I had an accident. Doctor with me, he was an intern. We would get calls and I got this call, the operator at the switchboard plugged in and contacted the driver of the ambulance so he could get the location. And I got this call. It was somebody that lived on Lincoln Street in the colored neighborhood off of Davis Avenue. So the caller said that the little girl had fallen out of a swing that was on a tree, tree limb. We think that she may have broken her back. I said all right, I'll get the doctor, intern that was practicing at City Hospital. They had interns those days. Well anyhow, I pulled up and got the doctor that was going to ride with me. He was from Washington, D.C.

Okay, we'll be there in a few minutes, hold on, be calm now. Hang up. Then I drove up and picked up the intern. Went this way on St. Anthony Street toward Springhill Avenue to go on to Catherine and then go Catherine to Davis Avenue. Well, I passed Dr. Purdue and Dr. Hinton. Passed them. They were in a car. They pulled aside when they heard the siren. That was us going by them.

And I just did get off of St. Anthony into Springhill Avenue, the widest street in Mobile. Well I was going, well anyhow get to Five Points, the street designated where the accident happened, and all of the sudden we passed two doctors that had just left the hospital, they pulled aside to give us the right of way and they saw this happen.

This car going east, we're going that way, clear, everything, all of a sudden this car, coming like this right in front of me. I went that way, kind of glance blow in front and it spun them around like that and the ambulance being like it was—over it went—and my arm was out the window. Gasoline spilling everywhere cause the tank was under the driver's seat. I remember this: they all ganged around real quick and all like that. Nobody smoke. Nobody smoking on account of the gasoline and they turned the ambulance back over on its four wheels. Then, this thumb was hanging way down there, and this arm was broken in the humerus and Dr. Hammond was a famous bone surgeon in those days. W. C. Hammond. He was great.

They wanted to take it off in the emergency room. Somebody said well we're gonna have to amputate Foster's arm. Dr. Hammond said no we're not. Gonna save it. Which they did. I watch them put a drill through that bone, and put a pin in it, put a clamp here, so they could tighten it up and pull this part here—try to get that where it would knit like that. But it knitted, done everything but right there and that's where it stopped, like that. I seen the picture of it that's why I can say what I was looking at. I only speak of mostly what I saw. I can think and tell the truth about it. Going by hearsay, what somebody else said, no. I don't go that route.

The ambulance was a Ford car. It was more of a truck than it was an ambulance those days. Top-heavy. The siren was up top. Yeah, you put it on, then you go on. Two red lights, that's all up front on the radiator out front. In those days, see that was 1936.

It's was according to what, the nature of the accident, whether it was a wreck, this that or what, somebody sick and needed an intern's attention, a doctor. Well, that was according to [the] nature of how quick you had to get there and get back to the hospital with the victim.

Well, I assisted them; I'd do anything and everything they would. Well, I hate to put it this way [hushed voice]. Very important. You know, we'd make a call. People didn't have much money in those days, no insurance or this that or what. They'd go out. And Dr. England, Frank England, and I had a call. Ms. Bessy Rencher was the truant officer and she called me. Go now, get a doctor and go down to this place way down in Oakdale. She said they didn't have anything and the lady is about to have a baby. I said yes ma'am. I got the location, got the doctor, we went out there. Frank England was on duty that day. It was nighttime, had a four-cell flashlight. At his orders and request, I held the flashlight while he delivered the baby. [Voice real soft] So, after. You see, your first time with something like that, that kind of seasons you a little bit. You never expected what you run into. I brought her and the baby to the hospital, see.

I made a call on the ambulance one time by myself. The doctors were busy at the hospital. This lady was pregnant, going to have a child. I got the call on it, so I went down to Oakdale, too. And coming back, Broad Street, slow, because she was ready at any time. You know there is a train track, you go over a little knob there. As I went over it like that, and the ambulance, it was a truck converted to an ambulance was what it was. I went over that. WAH WAH. I stopped and looked over and I said, oh my God! Nobody with me.

So I took it slow and I said be calm back there, now you stay calm back there, and I took it slow then. I got on into the, come in on the side of the old City Hospital, patients this that and everything and I told them what had happened. So naturally the doctors came out and nurses and assisted her on off and handled it. I get on the elevator—had to go up to the ground floor to the first level and they took it very easy, very careful. That was an incident that happened to me, that's why I can tell it and I speak the truth. I don't build up nothing.

At City Hospital they took care of mostly colored people and then the poor people, too.

That was covered by insurance. Back then that was the doctor's responsibility then. We would always comply with a doctor when they called. Well, the rich people, they wouldn't want to see the City ambulance with the red cross on it, saying City Ambulance and all. They'd get a private ambulance. Arthur Sermon had a private ambulance service in them days. Oh yes, they had private ambulances too. Well, Sermon was one of them. Arthur Sermon. He was one of the first ones to go that started in the private ambulance business.

Certain calls? Emergency calls? I'd put it. It's according; you can rate it just like you can a fire alarm. How many fire alarms come in a day at the fire station? Where there is a truck needed or a fire within the city limits or three-mile jurisdiction. And I put that as accordingly. It can't specifically be pinned down to answer accurately. We always responded to a practicing physician. See, they would call City Hospital. And then we'd go get the patient and bring him to the hospital. We had to get special permission to go outside the city limits. We could go anywhere within the city limits. But then in those days they didn't have no three-mile limit, or this, that or what they got now. See our fire trucks can go three miles outside the city limits on special call from someone of authority. Yes, ma'am.

Dr. P. J. Acker's office building, building of his office is still on Government Street, right by the courthouse, right next to the courthouse, that way. He was dean of the staff, the doctors' staff, and whenever a practicing physician called, we always responded. And if he wouldn't be able to give you a green light signal, put it that way, he'd leave it in charge with another one, well-known doctors like the one that I'm under now, he was well known cause he was a great surgeon. Dr. Don Oswalt. Yes, ma'am. The sisters are crazy about him. Cause he was a great, friendly. He's easy to get along with. In fact he would put his arm around a sister while walking down the hall or something. He was just a jolly, jolly, happy-go-lucky fellow. I'm telling you what I see, what I saw. I wouldn't say that if I didn't see it.

Well, when I was in the fire department, the ambulance would be passing the fire station going on calls. We'd hear the siren going, and there they'd go. And it would be passing, and we'd give them the eyeball. I don't know, I just, and the chief said, Foster? How'd you like to go drive that ambulance when Conniff wants to get off? I said, okay, Chief, I would. I was fascinated. Well, they're going to help somebody. I always felt sorry for somebody that needed help and have always rendered my assistance to help them; it's according to what the scene may be. You have a lot of put-ons, you know. A lot of people who would call that didn't need no attention. In those days, it wasn't, money wasn't free, and the population wasn't what it was now. If they had insurance, they'd be asked that question by the intern. And if they didn't, well that was a charity patient. See this was a city hospital. That's how they handled their business and well, I hate to put it this way. No, I better not mention, the majority, I'll put it even-even, white and colored, didn't have anything, this that or the other. But, we took our instructions; we never made our decisions unless we had authority, the boss. Sister Virginia, the head sister or a sister who is in charge of what ward, the OB ward, or whatever.

I remember one night I got this call to go to David and Eslavia Street, off of a Government for a severe earache. I said okay, I will. Got to the house. I said yessum, for an earache. The interns examined her on in the emergency room. Now somebody had told her to squirt some iodine in there. That was the worst thing that could ever happen. So they had to call a doctor whose office is on Bayou and Government, southwest corner. They called in this doctor that practices ear, eye, nose, and throat. His office and home was on, still is now, on southwest corner of Government and Bayou as you're going to the playground at the graveyard. He did the best he could, I didn't stay there and watch him, you know. But, I found out that she had put the iodine in there for the earache.

Well, if you investigated every emergency person that would come in on their own to get attention from an intern, a doctor, to get treated for whatever their problem may be, you'd be surprised. Anybody would be. All hours of the night and daytime, but nighttime mostly and it all would pick up. They would come in on their own. Course, you'd have to help them. Assist them. We were the City Hospital, owned and operated by the taxpayers.

They've got quarters back in the back for the ambulance driver. Telephone and a bed, just like a fireman, a police officer, you know. Ring the hospital number and the switchboard operator would call where we were. We would be asleep like the firemen do, back there. We worked 24 on and 24 off.

About home remedies? A policeman on the beat stopped and said, "Jim?" They called poppa Jim. Said, Jim, go out to Springhill and get red clay and bring couple of buckets with you. Bring it home, soak it in vinegar, and then get the oldest pillow that you have and cut it up where it'll be a foot square, 'bout like one of these, something similar to that. And put it in the oven and heat it and then put it on you. That's what they suggested. For rheumatism or slight injury, or ache or pain. That's what they used. Red clay, anywhere on the highway. It worked on poppa. Poppa had rheumatism in his arm; he was a longshoreman. He was working down at the foot of Dauphin Street. I'm going back now to 1914. I was a kid and I remembered that. Most of the country folks go for that too. People lived out in the country.

See, I was the only child by my mother. My mother finished St. Joseph's School. She went to New Orleans, practiced to be a nun. She didn't like it, she gave it up, came back to Mobile. That's when her and Poppa, 1885 or somewhere around there, got married. I told you about me bein born in Tampa; why we went to Tampa. But, this policeman, in the McNamara neighborhood; they called neighborhoods by names. He said you go out to Springhill and bring a couple of buckets of clay, get that red rich clay. He knew where a hill was that had the red rich clay, not just common clay, the real red rich clay. That particular clay, come back and make mud out of it with vinegar, the oldest pillow, use that for a pillowcase, could be like a bed pillow to be used and then you put it in the oven, let it get good and warm. Then apply it wherever your pain is. So help me, I'm speaking the truth. If you don't believe me, try it some time!

She would get an onion and peel it, chop it up and put it in the frying pan, a little butter and little lard mixed together, grease. Fry that onion then put it in jar, either with honey or molasses. Didn't have money enough to get honey, always more expensive than molasses was. Put the hot onion that you just fried in there. Let it cool off or whatever and use that for cough syrup when you had a cold. And then what saved my life when I was born. Dr. Hampton delivered me in Tampa. And I got off the track.

She'd get a piece of flannel, wring it out, put it on my chest, soaked it in camphorated oil. That odor from the camphorated oil, almost dry, and then put it on my chest. I had pneumonia. And the doctor that delivered me was our doctor named Dr. Hampton. I remember my mother telling me that a long time. He saved my life, hauled me over to the church where I was christened, a Catholic church. My mother was Catholic, my father was mostly Baptist, they say. But I never heard him talk about religion. But anyhow I remember momma telling me that in the olden days, treated me that way when I was not a year old yet. I would get a cold in my chest. Now that's the old times.

But they didn't, they didn't know what to prescribe. The doctors didn't even know how to write a prescription out in the olden days when you had a bad cold or cough or something. Sometimes you'd hit the jackpot with something like what I just said and it was favorable and I wouldn't repeat it if it hadn't been, but here I am now 87 years old and I was about to die with pneumonia. So my mother lived to be ripe age, so'd my daddy. Poppa died would have been 81 years on his birthday.

CHAPTER 5

Ernest G. DeBakey, MD (1910–2006)

Surgeon

Tulane University 1931

Tulane University Medical School 1939

Opened Mobile practice 1948

Interviewed on 6/2/94 at 84 years old

I was born and raised at Lake Charles, Louisiana. I decided to go into medicine because of a love for our doctor who was a general practitioner, a fellow by the name of Dr. Watson. And we used to go around with him on occasions where he would make calls and we got to know him real well and that's how my brother and I got interested in medicine.

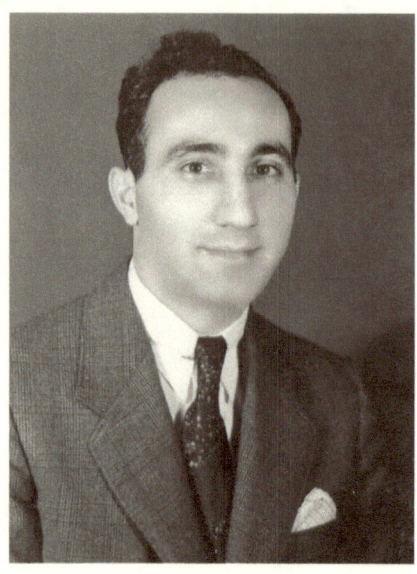

Ernest G. DeBakey, a medical student at Tulane University (December 1938)

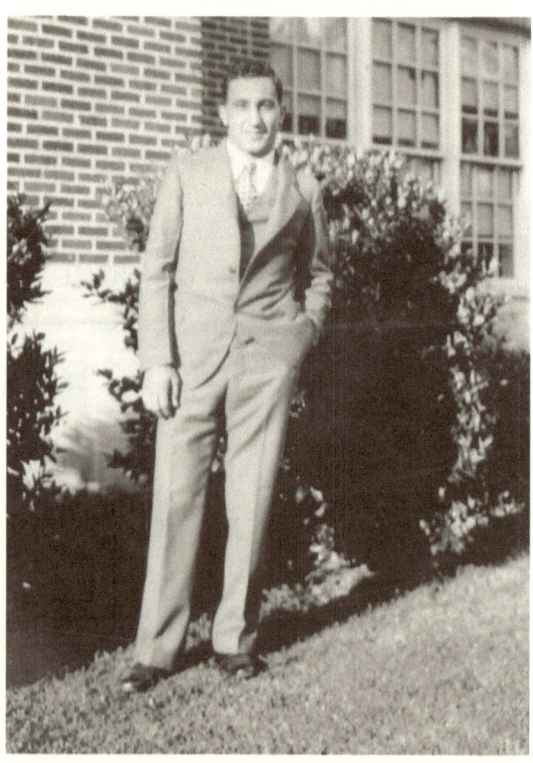

E.G. DeBakey outside Tulane University Medical School (1938)

After finishing high school I decided to go into pharmacy. So I went to Tulane and a two-year course in pharmacy. And after finishing I went back to Lake Charles and worked as a pharmacist for about four years. And then I saved enough money to go into medicine. So I went back to Tulane and entered the medical field in 1935. And I finished in 1939, a four-year course. And after finishing . . .

Well, first let me tell you, my senior year in medicine I decided to enlist in the Air Force Reserves. I wanted to go into flying. Yeah, I wanted to be a pilot. Well, I wanted to be both, a surgeon and a pilot, I guess. So anyway I graduated from Tulane in 1939 and interned at Charity Hospital for a year. And after completing that I went to Saint Louis as a first-year resident and I did mostly chest at Washington University. Came back to Tulane and finished that year as a resident. In 1943, I joined the active Air Force. They sent me to Randolph Field, at San Antonio, Texas, and {I} went through the fight surgeon's course which was several weeks. They taught me how to fly. It was a little PT19. Then I was sent to Stanford, Texas, a primary flying school for cadets, and I was there about I guess three or four months, maybe a little longer.

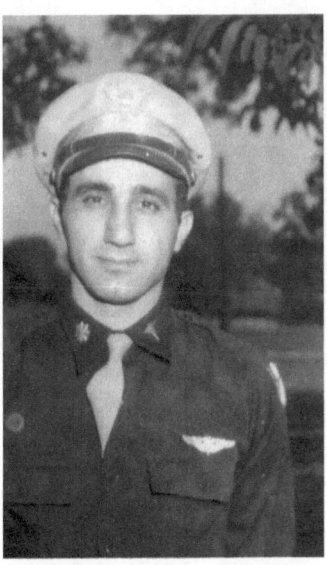

Major E.G. DeBakey (1944)

From there I went to Homestead, Florida, and got my orders to go to China: Burma Theater. This was a transport division of the Air Force and we were flying supplies from the Indian side into Main China. But anyway, it was not really an area where there was active enemy. We had a few Jap Zeros in the area but they were sort of a nuisance factor. There wasn't too much of a problem. I was there for about almost two years. We were along the Burma border and we had about five different locations. What we would do, we'd fly supplies from Calcutta, fly from these bases to Calcutta, and then fly over the Himalaya Mountains.

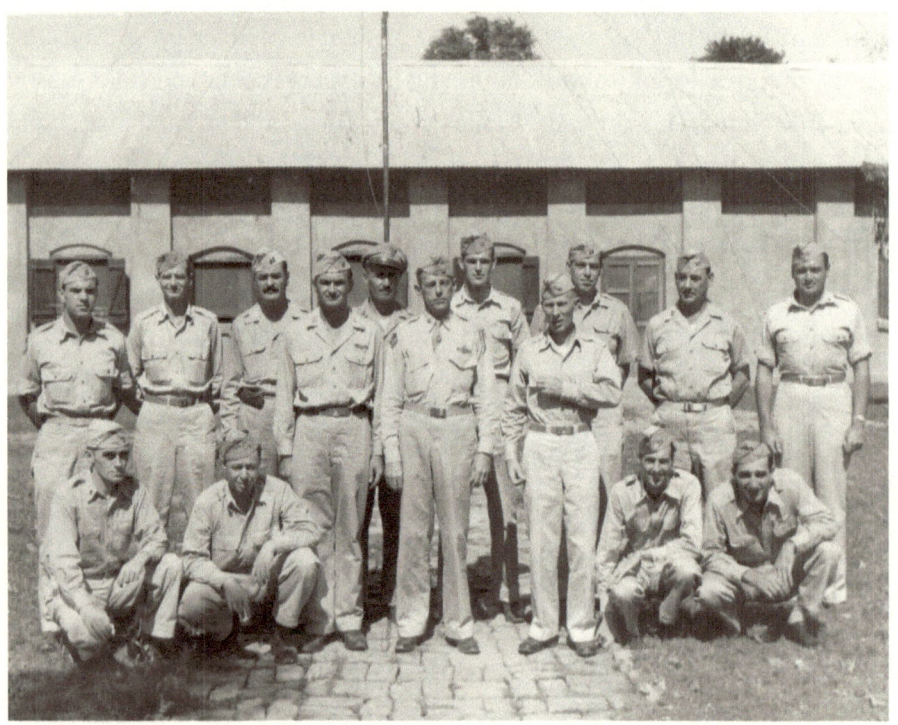

Taken at Lalmanirhat, India; Major DeBakey, flight surgeon, was in the first row far right (1944)

Then I came back to Homestead, Florida, and was asked to be transferred from the Air Force into the Medical Corps so that I could get back into surgery. Throughout my entire Air Force career I didn't do anything that amounted to anything. Then they transferred me and sent me to White

Sulfur Springs. I stayed there for about I guess about six or eight months. Then was discharged. I went back to Tulane and finished my residency in general surgery. And then I decided I was going to try to practice in New Orleans.

I finished my residency in '48. So then I wanted to practice in New Orleans. Dr. Ochsner offered me a job at Ochsner Clinic and my brother [Dr. Michael E. DeBakey, later of Houston] was there also at the Ochsner Clinic and I didn't think I wanted the clinic practice. Well, I couldn't very well stay in New Orleans without going to the Ochsner Clinic. I didn't feel like I could decline it and stay in New Orleans. Because of Dr. Ochsner, see.

So then I looked around and we just, one of the residents was Dr. McCafferty, who was from this area and he said what we ought to do is try to come over here. So we came over and looked it over. I wasn't too much impressed with it. I wasn't impressed with the medical community. There were not enough specialties (1948) and particularly what kind of discouraged me really was anesthesia. It was not very good. So then I went back to New Orleans and talked to one of the anesthesiologists who was graduating at the same time and asked him if he would go. He said we'll go take a look at it. He and I came over and looked at it. Well, he wasn't very much impressed with it either. And he said he didn't know whether he wanted to practice here or not. So we went back to New Orleans and talked it over and of course I was pushing him to go because I didn't want to stay in New Orleans. I wanted to stay in New Orleans but I didn't want to go to the Clinic. So anyway he came over and he decided that we would try it out anyway. That was Vernon [Dr. Balovich]. And it was kind of rough at first.

We came here in '48. Kimbrough was probably already here, I think. Dr. Wert I think had just arrived. John Day Peake was here. He was the only radiologist here. Dr. Wood was here. There was Dr. John Wilson. There was, well there were several of them doing surgery who were not surgeons, who were not trained surgeons. There was Dr. Frazier and there was Dr. Meeker and there was Dr. Taylor, Dr. Heiter. Let's see there was

Dr. Henderson, two Dr. Hendersons, brothers, and there was Dr. Warren Yem who was a board-certified surgeon.

We were trained. We earned our certification. Dr. Meeker and Dr. Frazier were grandfathered. They gave them their certificate without taking any examinations. We were the first ones required to be certified: Dr. Walker, Dr. Jim Donald, and myself.

Well, there were a few doctors who did not go to war. And they just controlled the County Medical Society. We had a hard time getting into the Society because they just blackballed us. They didn't want . . . competition. That's exactly right. That's what it boiled down to. And some of us, I really didn't have much trouble getting in. I got in after about two or three weeks. But the reason I got in, I think, there were very few surgeons here, see. Prior to the war the head of the Medical Society had issued a ban on accepting anybody into the Medical Society until the war was over and everybody had returned home. He said there would be a glut and he wanted to save the physician jobs for local men. And the others had more difficulty probably because they were internists and general practitioners, you see. So then it was fierce competition.

There was a lot of feuding going on: Meeker and Frazier. They were the two, probably the most important people here except there was a Dr. Purdue here in ENT [ear, nose, and throat] who was very powerful. But they had a very strong clique and they controlled the Society. And of course you know if you couldn't get into the Society, you probably couldn't get on the hospital staff, you see. So that's where the problems started.

Ms White-Spunner, who was a nurse, managed the Mobile Infirmary. Private. It was a private institute but it was founded on the basis of charity. Well, that's how it started, really, for Protestants and Jewish because the Catholics went to the other one. But anybody could come in. It was a nonreligious hospital, basically founded for charity. The charges at that time, I think it was a dollar a day for a room. And when I came here, which was years later after the hospital was founded, a private room was 12 dollars as I recall. It was on Spring Hill Avenue down at Catherine. That's Five Points. That's where the hospital was. I don't know exactly but I would think they probably had about maybe 75 beds or something like that.

Ms. White-Spunner was really the basis of the higher standards in the Mobile Infirmary. She, if it hadn't been for her there was no high standard here. And the nursing service was at the epitome the entire time she was here. The nursing service today is not anywhere near what the level that Ms. White-Spunner set for it. Now the reason for it, she was here every morning around six o'clock and she had a clipboard with her and she walked into every room every day. Every day. And she wanted to know from that patient what they were dissatisfied about and all that sort of stuff. And the nurses knew that and that's what set the high standard here. And when Ms. White-Spunner died that's when it went down. And I tried to get the administration here to do that same thing and they wouldn't listen to me.

After we got here and started practicing of course things were pretty difficult for us. I had my office in the Van Antwerp Building. There was a Dr. Sellers who was ENT and there was Dr. Warren Yem there who was in general surgery who was certified like I was and the rest of us that came about that time. And then there was Dr. Lester, in dermatology, and let's see who else. It's a small building. And there were some in the bank building. And Dr. Gilchrist was down there in the Merchant's Bank.

When I was in the Van Antwerp Building I had a little office and I divided the office. It was just small. It was very teeny. I only paid 65 dollars a month. And I didn't have an automobile so I rented an automobile. I rented an automobile for 132 dollars a month. And that was a brand-new Chevrolet. Four-door Chevrolet. I got all the gas I could use, oil, grease, and valet service if it rained for 132 dollars. And I got a new car every year. And I rented that car for about five years.

I came here with another surgeon from Tulane. He was a third-year. This was Dr. McCafferty. And we were partners. He's a good guy and a good surgeon and everything, but he didn't care to do too much work. Let me see, we came here in July. From July until January we took in 938 dollars. So anyway, we stayed together for about a couple of years and we decided to go our separate ways. We continued to help each other. But I just thought it would be better to strike out on my own so that's when it happened.

One of the interesting things I think you might want to know. About the time we came here we realized that there were a lot of people doing unnecessary surgery. They would do a laparotomy around one o'clock after they got through eating lunch and before going back to the office. So we decided—Dr. Howard Walker and Dr. Jim Donald and myself decided— to form the Surgery Committee. That's how the Surgery Committee got started.

We wanted to monitor the department of surgery to make sure that they were not doing unnecessary surgery. We thought that unnecessary surgery was certainly not the thing that surgeons should be doing. So then I mentioned the fact that I thought we ought to let the pathologist spearhead this because it will be a bloody battle probably if we were going to do it . . . I talked to Dr. Earl Wert and Dr. Howard Walker and Dr. Donald and the rest of us agreed that that would be the best thing to do to let Dr. Wert spearhead it. Well, he was responsible for pathology anyway. So they couldn't say anything about that. Well, he was happy to do it. Oh, yeah. And so we did it.

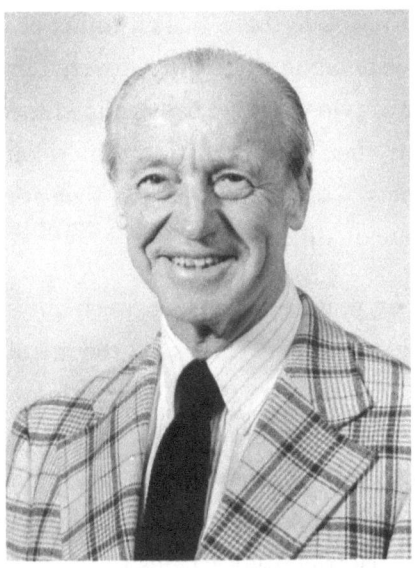

Dr. Earl Wert, pathologist, teacher, and director of tissue committees. From Dr. Webster: "Early on we had the best group of physicians who were meeting together with some regularity to discuss medicine ... He {Wert} began to lead those discussions . . . That was the first clinical teaching that was ever done in Mobile on any kind of regular basis and it was wonderful ... He was a good pathologist and is a good teacher, a very intelligent man. He did a great job of that, I want to say."

Did we get any opposition? Well, you see, you know, at that time the general practitioners were doing surgery, see, who were not trained in surgery but they were doing surgery. We did this to increase the quality. That was the only reason. It didn't mean anything to us. Not only to increase the quality, but to make sure that the people were being properly treated.

We saw a lot of unnecessary surgery—in all fields in surgery. We saw it in thyroid, we saw it in elsewhere: they would make an incision and . . . then close the incision. And we saw it in chest surgery. They'd . . . at that time they were doing some thoracoplastics which was not a very good operation. And they would make a little incision over a rib and they would cut out a little piece of the rib and call that thoracoplasty so we . . . Dr. Wert stopped all that. We put it on a very higher level.

When we came to Mobile there was an influx of internists and urologists. So you see we were being pretty well covered by the time I got here. Within the next year or two years we had certified specialists in practically all the other fields. By then the opposition to newcomers getting into the County Medical Society was about over. All that applied had no trouble getting in, if they were qualified.

During the earlier years relations between physicians was not very warm. But it was pretty nice between us, all the members who came in my time and right after. That was a very close relationship. Between the age groups there was still some problem. I think the loosing of power was probably worse in the field of surgery more so than medicine. I think there was a much closer feeling among those that came in at my time and the following years. There was a pretty friendly relationship, I think. Things changed a great deal and it was certainly a more pleasant atmosphere within say about four years after I had arrived.

When I came here I met a fellow through the bank, W. K. P. Wilson and Company. I had to have insurance on the automobile, etc., and so he sold me package coverage. For the office, and home and automobile. And then he said, well you need liability. I said, well I don't need liability. What do I need liability for? He said, well you ought to have it. I said well how much is it? He said well 75 dollars a year and that covered three hundred thousand dollars. So I said well if you say I need it I will. I didn't hear of any cases of liability when I came until about maybe 15 years later. There was a suit and I think it was a medical suit, if I'm not mistaken, but I think it was thrown out of court. That was the first one. Now subsequent to that, one of the surgeons, Dr. Guy Oswalt, was sued for an appendectomy. And I testified as a witness for him and it was a hung jury and then the suit was brought back and there was a local lawyer that tried it the first time so the second time it was this Belli from California. And he, Belli, came here but he did not try the case. One of his top men by the name of Ashe tried it and I testified for Dr. Oswalt and we won the case. Ashe, he was a brilliant lawyer. That's the first surgery case that I can recall.

The businesspeople: working and paper mill people got insurance. But the interesting thing about our time was that the patient was responsible for the insurance and for paying us. The patient paid us and the insurance paid the patient. And that's the way it should be now. See, I think the problem started when the doctor accepted the payments from the insurance company and relieved the patient of any responsibility. But they did that because they knew they were going to get paid. They were more interested in that than they were anything else.

Everything changed completely after insurance was available. I think . . . I think people go into medicine really because they love medicine and they know they can make a living. But then, it's not an easy way to make a living. The reimbursements are better than many other ways of making a living but I don't believe any doctor in my time went in because of the money. I don't think so.

The reason I think some people accept the idea doctors enter the field because the opportunity to make money is great is because today it's so expensive to get a medical education. By the time the doctor completes his graduation and becomes a doctor then he has about four or six years of postgraduate training. By that time he's married and has one or two or three children. Then he has to seek some way of recovering that debt. See. So what he does [is] he joins a group. He can't get enough money to open up an office to begin with and he naturally is concerned about his debt. You see. So I think that's where the people get the impression that he's a little bit more motivated by making the money than he is by treating patients. I can understand that, you see.

As a matter of fact I think that's where the reverence of patients began to disappear is when doctors joined groups where they don't have a direct relationship with anyone personally. It's, you know, no telling who you are going to see. And the doctor doesn't have the same feeling of devotion and trust that you would have as a solo practitioner.

The group practice started I think in the late fifties. Now, Dr. Hyman, urology, was solo when he came and all of the doctors were in solo practice when I got here. Those that were here before I got here.

I think there's competition in other businesses and in other fields but I don't think that that, I don't think its hatred, but I think it's kind of a slight disregard. For each other I guess. It's ego. It's the ego and status that probably develops that feeling. I don't know. But it has always been. Always will be I guess. When they are put on a salary, which I think all doctors are going to be in the not-too-distant future, I think it may be less of that.

Well, I think group practices developed because of the necessity for it. I think that those who were in solo practice had a tremendous clientele. And they couldn't take care of them. So they had to get someone to help them. I think that's what started it. It all began in internal medicine. And then you saw it start increasing where it covered dermatology. Now radiology years ago here in this hospital was only one person. That was Dr. John Day Peake. And then when it got beyond his ability then he brought in some help. Pathology started off as individuals, as solos. Dr. Wert was the only one here and they had one at Providence and then Wert brought in some help. He brought in Tommy Boudreau at that time and then brought in Montgomery and they did the same thing at Providence. But there was just one pathologist at both hospitals when I came in.

It was a big load when the documentation increased, you know. It was impossible to do that and to take care of patients. So you just had to have help. But group practice was the breakdown of the relationship between patient and doctor. See there's no direct relationship of long standing. You saw different doctors. You didn't see the same doctor every time you visited the doctor's office. And you didn't see it in surgery. Because it was felt that patients who are going to be operated on preferred one surgeon. They didn't accept someone else when they thought that this one surgeon that they had in mind was the best one for them, see? So . . . And that's basically true. So mostly patients stay with one surgeon. I think that's even true today. Even if there's a group, say A, B, and C, and an internist will recommend A, or B, or C. But they don't say go to that group and let them take care of you. They still refer to one individual in surgery, and I guess when someone's operated on they feel a little bit more concerned than taking a medication. And so they want somebody who they believe has had a good reputation. I think when a doctor refers a patient to a certain doctor they feel confident and secure with that doctor's referral. They think he knows all about him, so I'm going to accept that.

I think faith in ability has a great deal to do with healing. I think it has a great deal to do with it. If you have confidence in someone, then the trust that you develop is enough for the individual to accept whatever that doctor tells them. If there's no trust then they're not going to accept the doctor's treatment. I don't think there's any question about that. You see, if you will just look back in the days of herbal medicine, you see, if that herb doctor told you that this herb is more valuable for you and is going to help you more than another herb, you're going to take that herb that that doctor recommends. It's basically the trust that you can develop with a patient and a doctor. I think it's 100 percent of the healing. Oh, yeah.

My best time to practice was over the last say thirty years: sixties to the nineties. And I think that will continue. You see, when I began my career we were doing a lot of surgery that we don't do today because of the improvement in medical care. It's rare to operate on someone for an ulcer anymore. It's just rare to operate on thyroids anymore unless it's a malignancy, you see. There were many improvements there that eliminated a great deal of surgical trauma.

CHAPTER 6

Socrates Nicholas Rumpanos, MD (1914–2007)

Surgeon

University of Alabama 1933

University of Alabama 1935

Duke Medical School 1937

Opened Mobile practice 1940

Interviewed on 5/27/94 and 5/31/94 at 80 years old

Why medical school? That's an odd story. When I finished high school my older brother that was two years ahead of me had been working with the county civil engineers. When I finished high school, Murphy (Mobile), the day after the graduation exercise we went back home. Pop asked me did I want to go to college. He said I'm going to send Gus—he saved enough money to go. This is Depression years, this is 1930. He said your Uncle George and myself can help get you up there, too. I said, sure I want to go. I hadn't given it a thought. He said, what are you going to study? He said Gus is going to study electrical engineering. I said I don't know, since it's a shock. He said, why don't you study medicine? And I said okay. That was it. I think that was always his ambition, was to study medicine. I was 16. I had no plans whatsoever to go to college.

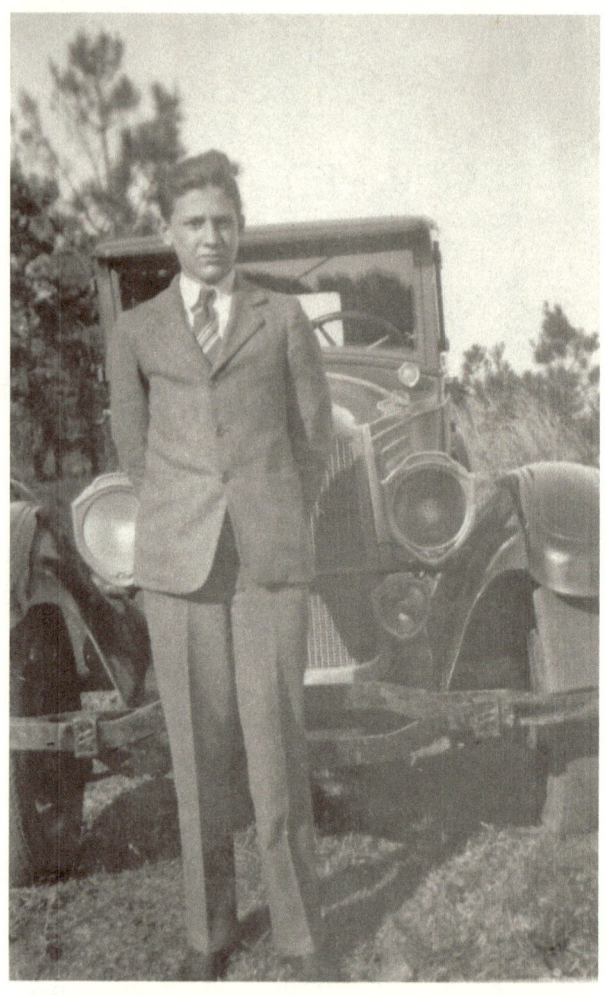

Socrates N. Rumpanos (at 15, 1929)

We went to the University of Alabama for undergraduate work. Alabama only had a two-year medical school then. I got an AB in three years and one summer and then I went on to med school for two years in Tuscaloosa and transferred to Duke. We would come home on weekends and would work. Papa would lay off somebody on Friday nights and we would work all day Saturday and make twenty-five bucks apiece and go back up. We had an old Hudson automobile that would go anywhere; old big Hudson touring car.

Then off to Duke for medical school for the last two years. Alabama first for two years, then we had to transfer.

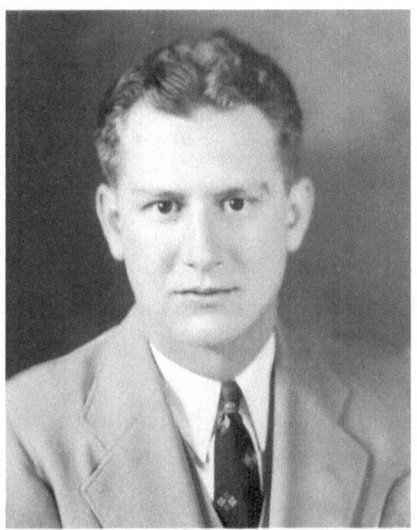

Socrates N, Rumpanos (at 21) graduating University of Alabama (1935)

Of course, everybody at Alabama wanted to transfer to Tulane because it was a closer school and the cheapest. Eighteen of us applied. It's very dense, very fixed in my mind. Then Tulane told the faculty to pick five. That was all they could take. Well I was one of the five that was picked and was real happy! When school was out in June we all usually went to see the dean and tell him good-bye and thank you. He said, well, Rumpanos, where are you going to school? I said Tulane and he shuffled some papers and he said, no, you're not. I said, what do you mean? I said I was picked and was told that. He said, yeah, but you were sick. I missed a month. I got jaundice, undiagnosed jaundice, and spent a month in the hospital up there. But my roommate helped me catch up and, in fact, I made the best grades I ever made because I was too damn sick to play.

He said we've given your place to someone from Butler County, a politician's son from up there. And I said well, hell, I've got to go somewhere. He said, "Well I used to be dean up at Tennessee," he said, "Would you mind going there?" I said no I'll go anywhere. He said well, I'll get you in up there. I took his word for it and I said okay and walked out. A month later I hadn't heard from him and I called him and no answer. Two months later, this was July; I went up there because he wouldn't return my calls. The secretary told me, well I've given him the message was all she would tell me. I went up there and ran him down at his home. I was kind of hot. And he told me that they didn't have any openings there. He said he had tried everywhere, so I really felt let down. So I called Frank Boykin who was a personal friend and everything. Frank was in Congress then. He was a representative. I told him what had happened and he said oh, I'll make them take you. I'll make them take you! I found out later that he was the one that made the Dean put that Butler boy in my place, but he didn't tell me that.

Luckily one of the instructors we had, who was from Duke, had taken a summer job there to make a little money teaching physical diagnosis. He just happened to be in Tuscaloosa for a semester teaching because his home was in Birmingham. He has a brother that was a urologist in Birmingham. He was from Clanton, Alabama, originally, but he ended up professor of dermatology at Duke. He taught most of the dermatologists in this part of the country. He called me. We had two men going to Duke and one of them was my old roommate and one of them was a boy from Baton Rouge.

When he called me I was down at Tarpon Springs on a wild party. Golly, there's a place, a hotel down there that . . . Oh, gosh, it would put the Grand Hotel here to shame. Gee it was a beautiful place. Pop called and said you've got a telegram here. He said, do you want me to read it to you? It has been here a couple of days. He said it's from a Dr. Callaway in Durham, North Carolina, and he said if you want to come to Duke, come on up and work as an extern. He said you can start the fall quarter in September. Gosh, all I had was the month of August and I had to go up there and work one month. Man, I thanked that man the rest of my life! And that's how I got to Duke.

After Duke I went to Baltimore and interned on surgery at City Hospital, and then I went to the University of Maryland on surgery. I was the chief of surgery's assistant. It was really a residency thing. It was a brand-new hospital. The University of Maryland was an old school, but they had opened up a new hospital and at City Hospital we had both a Hopkins staff and a University of Maryland staff. Gosh, it was ten thousand beds.

I stayed on with Dr. Shipley as his assistant. Of course he gave me stuff ahead of the residents, the official residents, so I was in hot water all the time with them. They had a resident staff, but it was all new to them and Shipley wanted someone he could depend on. It made the residents mad because I got to do all of Shipley's work. I assisted him. Stuff that he didn't want to do he'd let me do. Either he'd help me or I'd find someone to help me. I was going to stay on with him for the equivalent to a full-term residency but the medical service took control of the house staff the following year. The internists, they hated surgeons. Shipley had me as his first assistant and nobody else on the staff had a first assistant, they had to use just the house staff, so I was just a redheaded stepchild. I knew I was going to get fired and so I would have to go over and start from the bottom up with the staff. We knew then, too, that the war was coming on. Stuff was hot. This was '39. I finished at Duke in '37. We knew the war was coming on and they were kind of recruiting for the war. Meanwhile I got married—she was Shipley's nurse!

I called Mobile—they were always having trouble getting physicians. The City Hospital had never been accredited for AMA internships even. That's how backward we were then. I came down. Dr. Eddings from up in Peterman, Alabama, had been at Callaway's and knew he was going to have to do a lot of OB in his country practice, so he had called from Birmingham and wanted to come down. There were the three physicians that they ordinarily took as interns at City Hospital. One of them was from what they called a grade-B medical school who was a good doctor but he came from a real underrated school and he didn't even know whether he was going to get accredited for a license. There were two other guys: a two-year man, a Mobile boy, who came home for another year, and another guy. Plus a boy who ended up over in Mississippi practicing somewhere. There was six of us. They didn't last long. The fellow in Mississippi left first to go into private practice.

Married Gertrude in '38. Brought her down here with me while I joined the other men at the City Hospital to try to get them an organized staff because they had no services and no accreditation. It was just an old general hospital. Doctors in town would go out there and operate and all. They all put in a year there and then went on in to practice. Pretty primitive. That's what it was. We wanted to get them organized into medicine, surgery and OB, and orthopedics. It was just us. We were paid 75 dollars a month by the city and county. There wasn't a whole lot to it. The Sisters realized the problem was that they didn't have any accreditation. They knew all of us were going to go eventually into practice, most of us in Mobile, or we thought so. But one left right away; he got a big offer in Pascagoula, then another went to Pensacola to go in practice.

Frankly, I didn't look too far in the future because I knew—we all knew—from talking—that we were going to be in the service before too long. We weren't trying to prolong it but they weren't recruiting medical people that much. Even though they knew they were going to need them, they did very, very little recruiting. They did a lot of talking that they were going to need doctors, that they were going to need nurses and all this and that. I came home with the knowing that I would eventually be in the service. I thought I could help out here and get acquainted with the doctors

It was a lot of fun over there at the City Hospital. We worked hard. We would not let a patient go to a bed without a history and physical. That was the big thing. Inspectors make rounds and there have to be histories and physicals on the charts and stuff like that. And we would have to ride the ambulance . . . Foster can tell you that. You know they applied for accreditation every few months. Even though we had orthopedic beds and we had surgery beds and medical beds on the ward, there were no services. Whoever was on duty that day looked after them. You weren't assigned surgery; you weren't even classified as medical or surgeon. Everybody did everything. But we got that place accredited. It was fun. We worked 20 hours a day but we still had fun. We didn't have but maybe 150 beds, but even then that's a lot of people. We had surgery every day, we had babies every day, and we had outpatient clinics to run. And trauma. We worked hard.

Made 75 dollars a month. Then they held out 25 dollars. Gave us room and board. Dr. Acker was the king bee of medicine in those days. After everybody left he made them hold out 25 dollars a month on the three of us so we wouldn't leave. I hated that man with a passion, too. I got to where I liked him.

I went into practice in '40. I went downtown and shared an office with a dentist in the Park Building. I was above my daddy's store so I would go down and eat. Frank Boykin's office was right there with us on the same floor. I took a little girl that was just finished training as a secretary and she did everything. That was the only assistant I had. I didn't have much work anyhow. No. I went out to the Mobile Infirmary and examined and wrote histories and physicals for one hundred dollars a month to kind of feed my wife. And what little practice I had I think I made 58 dollars the first month and I had to pay my house loan and my bills. I saw patients in the office and made house calls. I assisted whenever they would ask me to help them in surgery. I was a ghost surgeon a couple of times. A couple of them, all they did was make the incision and sit there and talk while you did it. And then all you'd get was a 25-dollar assistant fee out of it and he'd get the big fee. Some of them weren't able to do the procedure they had scheduled and thought they needed help. They had some crummy doctors in those days. You talk about ghost; they'd get us to do their operating for them!

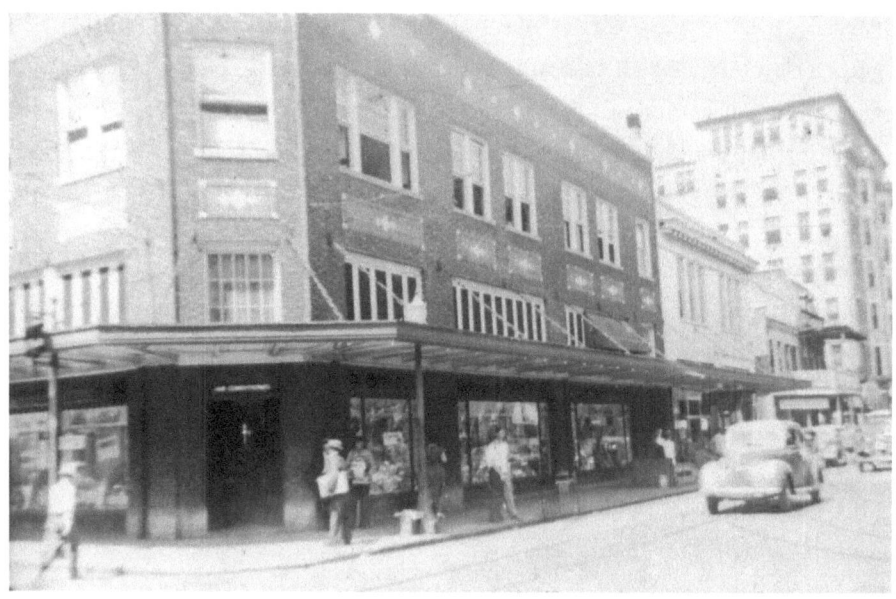

Dr. Rumpanos opened his Mobile practice in 1940 in an office on the second floor, above his father's fruit stand store, where he went to lunch daily.

There were some good men practicing medicine. But those guys that were here before the war, their intentions were good, but their skills were not necessary. Even after the war they still had a lot of influence . . . We didn't have any blacks in the medical society when I first got in it. But they also weren't applying—they knew better than to apply. There was enough of the older fellows in there and they were going to get blackballed. So they just stayed out and everybody got along fine with them in practice. They couldn't admit to the hospitals. The only place they could send anybody to was the City Hospital. Then they couldn't look after them after they got them there. They had to turn them over to the staff.

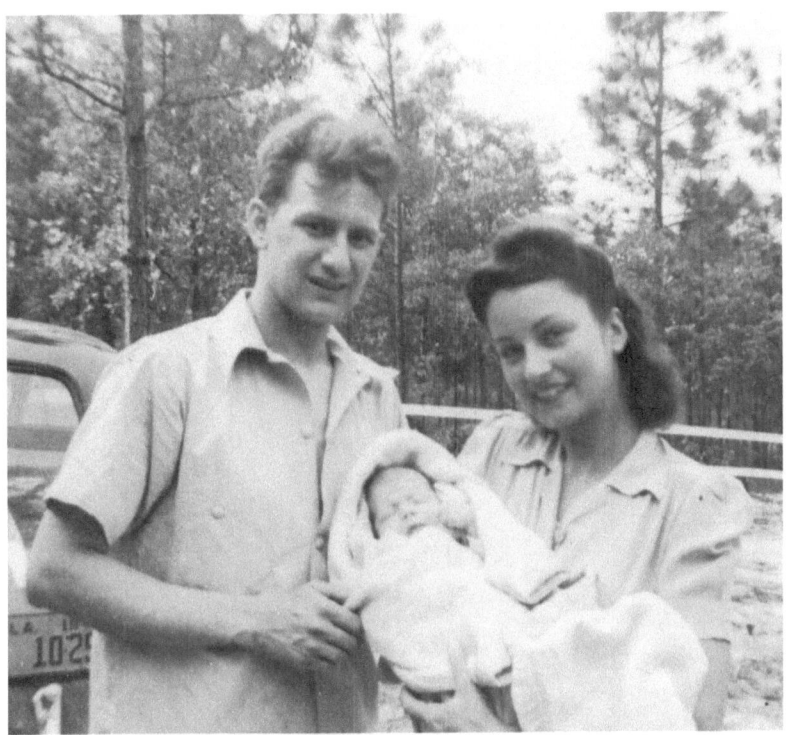

Dr. Socrates Rumpanos, wife Gert, and daughter Jean in 1941

Things had picked up a lot for me then. I had been helping Dr. Frazier and Meeker and they had a lot of surgery, but they were on the wrong side of the political fence. Yeah. I was helping them then and really picking up a lot because I wanted to do surgery. That's all I had done in Baltimore. Down here I had to do everything so I got the reputation of having done everything and that was only because I had to. Then when the war started I went to New Orleans to get into the Navy; went way before Christmas because I think it was the seventh of December when they bombed Pearl Harbor and they told me I'd get orders within a month.

I came home and closed the office and everything; told them I would pay one girl to stay there six months to collect bills and whatever. I passed the word around I was just going to be available to help assisting and everything. It's a crazy story. I didn't want to leave anybody real sick, with no one specific to look after them. And I sat around and sat around and

nothing happened. I'd call them up and they would say it was being proc-
essed. Called Frank Boykin again and tell him I'd applied to get in the
Navy and they had accepted me but that I hadn't gotten orders. Joe Little:
he'd gotten in the Army as a major. He was only eligible as a lieutenant in
the Navy. I was going in as a JG {lieutenant junior grade} because I wasn't
but 27 years old, and Boykin said he would check. That was in December.
I think it wasn't until June that I got word that the reason that the Navy
didn't give me a Navy commission was that I was a reserve officer in the
Army Coast Artillery. I'd forgotten I'd taken ROTC at the university.

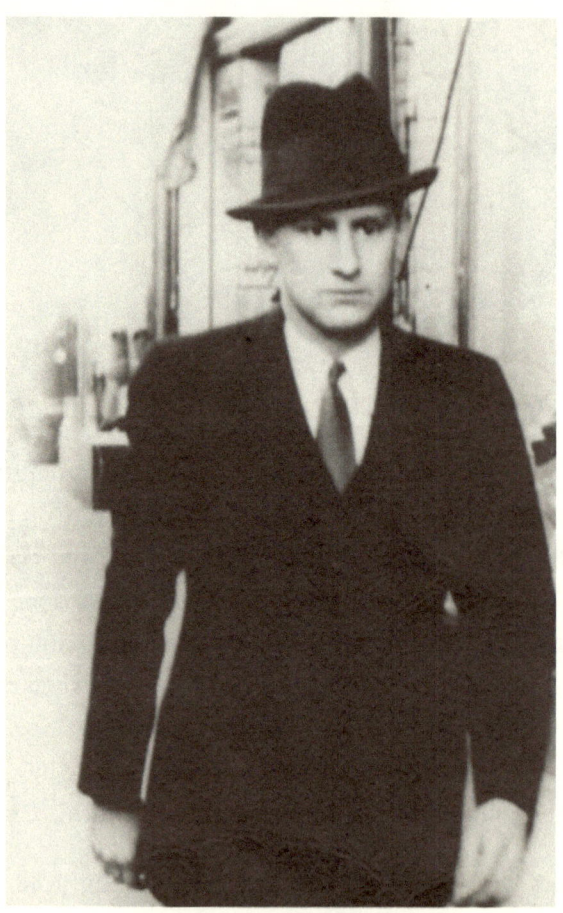

Dr. Rumpanos (1941)

I told them no, I didn't want to be in the Coast Artillery! I was a doctor. I wanted to be Navy but they never sent me orders. There I was—all this time I could have been making big money: everybody was gone. Finally I got that transfer and I got my orders. Joe Little had already gone. Frazier had gone and Meeker had gone. Amandola was still here and Amandola made big money surgically; and Dr. Heiter was here and Charlie Rutherford, big Charlie. They were doing all the surgery. Oh, he's a swell guy. And Heiter was a dream. Heiter was a love. Everybody was crazy about him. They deserved it.

But there was also old man P. M. J. Acker. He thought he was the king because he used to be a teacher at the old medical school when it was here in Mobile. And he and Dr. G. O. Seagrest were the biggest rivals you've ever seen. There was a picture of the City Hospital staff and they're standing with their backs to each other. They wouldn't even look at each other. That's why they're turned outward—they hated each other with a passion. They got jealous of each other. Thinking they were better than the other.

The Navy didn't send me anywhere. That was the thing. I thought I would be in for a couple of weeks' indoctrination and then I'd get a shift. They put me in school, back in school. Not for a few weeks like we thought, for a whole damn year at the Bethesda Naval Medical Center in Maryland. Right outside of D.C. Really it was biological warfare. It was a secret type thing. They only trained one class. There was 69 of us started and only 29 graduated. We had exams every week and they'd cut—bring the ax in. It was the hardest damn work I've ever done in my whole life! We studied warfare. It was bacteria, stuff that would kill you, stuff that would make you so damn sick. We had evidence. It was a real, real, real interesting course, I mean it . . . Our professors and most of the class were big shot professors from Yale and Harvard, bacteriologists and physicists and whatnot. They were all lieutenants and lieutenant commanders. They were six JGs. They had to fill up the class. That's what happened. We just got the commission. We just happened to be the six guys who filled up the class. I spent a damn year locked in. We didn't know from one day to the other whether we were going to be there because they swung active.

We grew leprosy bugs. We grew TB bugs. Real real dangerous stuff: all the bacteria that causes diarrhea. We had evidence of Japanese learning . . . oh gosh, it's all coming back to me. There was a liver fluke that caused filariasis. It caused all the leg sweating and edemas in the Marines on these islands. The Japanese found out there was a pig that was an intermediate host, the pig that could carry it and the kids would kill the wild pigs on the island and eat them and they'd get this damn liver thing. The Japanese didn't try to kill them, they just tried to put them out of business. One whole Marine division, ten or fifteen thousand, was put out of commission on one particular island from the liver fluke. They got their legs and everything swollen.

One of our crew—after we graduated they had divided us up into units and each Marine division took one of our units with them and each naval district got one of our units. I came to Pensacola and worked for a year on account of the guy that was my boss. Down in Pensacola—after a year in Bethesda—most of our units went out. Went out with the Marines when they were doing their island hopping and we'd get reports back. One of them went crazy: they put him on an island to check and he went nuts because the submarine forgot to pick him up. Apparently the submarine got lost. One of our doctors. When they found him they said he was completely nuts. Up in a tree like a damn monkey and they couldn't get him down. They think that what happened was the submarine that was supposed to pick him up got sunk or got lost or something.

When I was in Pensacola we had evidence of the chemical warfare. They showed us movies just like the old newsreels here of the Japanese launching these paper balloons to try to bomb the United States. When they hit the Rockies they'd come over at forty thousand feet. The Rockies would separate them and they'd either go up to Canada or down to Mexico. Some of them killed some kids in Canada when the balloon came down. They had what they called antipersonnel bombs on them. What we were looking for was a bacterium, because the Japs had used them against the Chinese with two particular bacteria.

One was called rendafess, which kills chickens and ducks and whatnot. The other was hoof-and-mouth disease, actinomycosis, which kills off the animals. So they were trying to starve the Chinese out with them. We had captured movies of them launching; we could see the serial numbers of these paper balloons coming over here to America and all of them hitting the West Coast. We'd get reports on them every week—what was happening. Well they finally figured out how to clear the Rockies. Their spies over here were telling them—that's how complicated the damn course was. It was so damn interesting time flew by like that! When they started clearing the Rockies some of the balloons came down around Detroit. They were trying to hit the factories there where they were building the tanks. I don't think they had bacteria in them. I think they were just trying to see if they could get it over here.

On several of those they had a box about the size of a shoebox with agar in them, which is a culture material. But we could never recover any bacteria. When they started hitting Detroit, they called us all. They sent me to Philadelphia and then we had a big conference on Governors Island with the Army because they had similar units. We even cultured the paper that the balloons were made out of to see if they could be hiding in there. But we never found any bacteria on any of those that cleared the Rockies. The only thing I ever saw in public on that was an article in an engineering magazine. I brought it over here one day to show it to Dr. Wert. Wert knew a couple of the guys that were in my class because they were pathologists and bacteriologists and all. We had a guy named Fobegale who was head of bacteriology at Yale and he was the smartest man I've ever known. Actually he was the one who organized this thing. We covered a 178-page book of calculus in five days. Took an exam on it. We covered some weather stuff that, hell, these weather people said my God, that's two years' work! We covered it in two weeks. Yeah, we learned how to read the balloons. When they'd drop to thirty thousand feet they would light up like a firecracker and cut loose the sandbag and the balloons would shoot back up. We had it figured out how they did it but none of that ever came out in the damn war trials. That's what made us mad.

When we were in Philadelphia we had a couple of meetings over on Governors Island. It was the damnedest thing I've ever seen. They had the admirals and generals up front and then they had a great huge building. The JGs . . . We were in the backstage and we didn't even have seats because we were the ones doing all the work. And if you took notes, there were Marines and MPs at the door that took your notes away from you when you went out. Here our own people! I had looked up this admiral who was a friend of Dr. Meeker's that I knew was going to be there. I was up in his hotel room having a drink with him; a knock on the door and there were two shore patrol officers and they said admiral we understand you walked out with your notes. He refused to give them to the shore patrol that were at the door. He said, yes, he wanted to read them before I destroyed them. He said I wanted to read over them and he said I didn't have time. I had my ride there. We had to go by boat because we were on an island. They said, well where are they now? We'd like to have them. He said in the East River, I flushed them down the commode. They took his word for it. He read the notes over and just flushed them.

When I stayed in Philadelphia I brought Gert and we had a second daughter by then, brought her up there and rented a house. She didn't like Philly even though her home was in Baltimore. She just stayed six months and came on home. When the war was over I didn't have enough time overseas duty to get out on points. You had to have a certain amount and they were using all the doctors to do the examination of everybody that was being discharged. Hell, I spent almost an extra year just doing nothing but physical exams. One of our classmates had taken over head of the biological warfare department and he was stationed in Texas. It was coded. There was just a bunch of letters. But it was really biological warfare. He took over head of it and called me up and said, Soc, you want to go home? I said you're damn right I do. He said "You're not going to be able to get out. They're going to keep us in the reserves in case we have another war or anything. We'll be teachers in the same stuff." He said, "I can put you some orders and you can go on home, but you're going to have to stay in the reserves." I didn't get out of the Navy until I was 72 years old [1986]. I tried to get in the Navy Reserves because they get promotions and all.

They were afraid we would lose our identity as biological warfare experts. I got one promotion. I went from lieutenant JG to lieutenant. That was all. For 40 years. I asked them if there was anything I could do if I were going to have to stay in—to get a promotion. They said no, just got to be available on call. Never got called. I have a brother who is a dentist. Went in as a lieutenant and in nine years he was a four-striper, which is a full colonel. I got kicked around but I had fun. I don't regret a minute of it.

I would like to say something about the way after the war how things really picked up. Yeah, before the war everybody was unfriendly to each other. They were, I mean, even socially they didn't speak to each other. It was . . . No, the war made a big difference. When we got ready to leave a guy named Dr. Woodruff from Anniston came down here and recruited as many doctors as he could for the government. That was his job. He was an officer, a reserve officer. Locally, Dr. S. J. Walker's daddy was a character—he was the coroner. He was the official coroner and he had a lot of power because the coroner is the only guy that can arrest the sheriff. He outranks the sheriff in politics. He made a motion not to accept any more members to the medical society until after all of us got drafted.

He got mad at Woodruff. For leaving the town depleted, because it left very few of them here. Other than you know a few old men because I think Amandola and Speedy Brown were about the only two that were underage and ineligible for the draft. He made a motion not to accept any more members. And then some lady doctor came in here. I forgot what her name was. I never did know her. They blackballed her. She took it to court and got in. So frankly that got everybody together more than anything else. And it wasn't the woman. It was the fact that he had passed the motion and the medical society would not take any more in until we got back, not that it mattered. It was just Dr. Walker being angry, but not at the lady. I was there for the vote. Walker really did some politicking to get that thing pushed. I didn't vote on it. When they took a vote to see about restricting any new members, I said hell, I'm not going to be here anyhow so why should I put my neck out and have somebody get mad at me for blackballing her. It was tough going. And then the lawsuit got them together and they said we're damn fools to stay in the public eye blackballing a qualified person.

Oh there was still some hard feelings. For instance . . . the only private hospital I could get on was the Mobile Infirmary, but I agreed to write the histories and physicals . . . one hundred dollars a month, no matter how many patients. That was the only hospital that accepted my application. I don't know why. I helped get the accreditation at City Hospital and I could go in there and help, but I couldn't admit. At the Providence and City Hospital I applied to get on in surgery because that's what I wanted to do and I had real good exposure to surgery when I was in biological warfare. Every station I had I knew the surgeons. Dr. Meeker was chief at Pensacola and I worked with him. He gave me plenty of work to do. I had the time to do it because I had my people running the lab and I didn't have anything to do. And the same way in Philadelphia: Dr. Meeker told me who to look up.

When I did get on in the service the only thing available was urology and proctology, and I didn't want any proctology, so I took the urology. Dr. Frazier was chief of it then. He and Tommy Boudreau were the only two decent urologists in town. Boudreau was one of the best urologists you've ever seen. A prince of a guy. Frazier got me on over at the City Hospital in urology and I eventually got transferred to surgery. I ended up chief of staff over there, back in the forties. I showed them. Show you how popular I was when I was chief of staff, and not just surgical, the whole damn works—I had monthly meetings and you know how many of my own meetings I got invited to? Zero. Sister would set the date. The Sisters, the nuns ran the damn thing and they didn't want the physicians to have anything to do with it. All they had had were yes-men up until the time I got elected by the staff. But the doctors were there. We were trying to get to have something to say about the way things were run. This is so different from the way it has been in the last 30 years.

I noticed a change in quality of health care and the quality of services— I'll tell you, a lot of it started when Blue Cross was available. See we have a long time there with nothing like that except for industrial cases. They were the only ones that were covered. But when Blue Cross came in here, when you knew you were going to get a little money, a little bit more attention was paid to it. Blue Cross wasn't paying everything. We'd bill what we wanted to and if we wanted to accept it we did, but it wasn't mandatory, it was just a percentage.

We tried to get set fees because Blue Cross asked us to, but we couldn't get physicians to agree. I asked them, begged them. We tried, because I was president of the county medical society, too. I said, let's set a fee. Put it in the safety deposit box somewhere. So when Blue Cross and other insurance companies approach us and ask us what the fee is for this area, because that's what they went on, we can open up the box and show it to them. You don't have to agree to it but we got what we all think is an average fee, like one hundred dollars for an appendicitis, two hundred dollars for a gallbladder, anything like, just have something in writing. They wouldn't do it. So Blue Cross took advantage of us and so did Aetna and all these other insurance companies. They said, we'll pay so much for an appendicitis. The physicians didn't give a damn. They figured they could bill them for the rest. They very seldom got paid. Very few of them did. They just didn't want to agree with each other. You could not get doctors to agree.

Now what happened after they finally came to a fixed fee, Blue Cross and the other insurances that were selling hospital insurance had your fee. Well, hell, if you wanted to charge one hundred dollars for an appendicitis, you can't charge any more than that. A young man comes along and charges 250 dollars for an appendicitis. Well that's his starting fee. They'll pay him 250 dollars but they're only going to pay us one hundred dollars, because that's all you've ever charged and we got caught with all that. Blue Cross had gone back and looked at the actual billing records. They knew exactly what you charged . . . We all got stuck, the old-timers did. I had a youngster the other day say hell he wouldn't do an appendicitis for less than 1,100 dollars. He couldn't live and that's what they are getting these days. Anesthesia probably gets eight hundred dollars. They used to get 25 dollars at most for an appendicitis. It's absolutely insane.

These youngsters came in here and they were getting paid to intern. I think the starting salary for internships was eight thousand dollars. Residencies these days get anywhere from eighteen thousand dollars to twenty thousand dollars, and they were used to making money. Residents, whoever organized interns and residents, sure did them a favor. They're not going to go into practice without knowing that they're going to be able to get big money. It's strictly business now. I don't know when it changed, but I sure hated to see it. I'm glad I'm out of it. I noticed a change mainly when the insurances came along and said by gosh we'll pay 100 percent. Some of the docs said, very few said, that's more than I would charge. But look at your eye people, gosh, what they get for cataracts. They used to do cataracts for one hundred dollars and do 20 a day; three and four thousand dollars.

Things started changing when insurance began to be available. The insurances are fine as far as I'm concerned to help people. But who is going to pay all these people and all the administration it's going to take to run the things? The government is taking over but they're doing it in steps. If a guy in one area was doing too many gallbladders he has to quit doing only a certain number and somebody else had to do them. We had worked like hell to get them where we could operate 24 hours a day. We did it for the longest and it was very, very successful. The Mobile Infirmary got to be the best, biggest operating room in this part of the country and all of a sudden they said no, you couldn't do that anymore.

I don't know what happened. If we wanted to do a gallbladder at midnight we could do it. Nobody wanted to particularly, but if they couldn't get it on the day schedule then we could go ahead and do it instead of having to wait. Go up there now. In fact the last time I was up there visiting one of the head honchos, some physician wanted to do something: "Just tell him he'll have to get in line," before they'd find him a room. The rooms were empty. They just didn't have the help to do it and they didn't want to call in the help to do it. Trying to hold expenses down.

Most of the youngsters as they would come in, have been real good men. We haven't had the alcoholics we used to have a couple years ago that were real bad and we had to watch them, and couldn't . . . Got them off the staff. We did that. It was fun when everybody got along.

When we were building the Mobile Infirmary Mr. Bedsole took all our names and divided into teams. The banks had all gotten together with him and given him a list of about what everybody had and he told us how much to ask everybody for. Frank England, Joe Little, and myself had one of the teams and gosh we had them down for anywhere from five hundred dollars over a five-year period up to twenty-five thousand dollars. Bedsole got all the information but we didn't know it. What incomes they had or what. They had one guy here that had come during the war and he was in country practice. Nobody knew much about him yet. He built up a big practice because he was available for ob-gyn and he just called himself that. All he was doing was country practice before that. I don't think he had any specific training, so we went to see him because we had him down for five hundred dollars, because nobody knew anything about him locally.

We went in there and told him we got you down for five. We figured he knew what we were going ask for, because we had called and made an appointment with him. Well, but he said you could spread that over a five-year period. He said to tell you the truth I'd like to pay it in a lump sum because I've had a good year on the cotton market. So we said that would be all right. So he wrote us out a check for five thousand dollars. We looked at him. He said well I wish I had a drink for you gentlemen, I'd offer it to you. I said I happen to have some out in the car. We were only going to hit him for five hundred dollars! When we told him five he took it for five thousand so we took his check for five thousand dollars. We found out later that he had an uncle that was a cotton broker in New Orleans and he had given him some tips and he had made a fortune on the cotton market that particular year!

Ms. White-Spunner was one of the greatest women that ever walked. I have every respect in the world for her. She knew every patient in the house.

She saw every one of them every day. She was the administrator. When Bramlett came in she told us, she called about nine of us together and said, now listen, Mr. McRae from the bank wants Bramlett out here. She said now don't y'all run him off. He was her understudy. He had no hospital experience whatsoever other than his daddy being a doctor in Mississippi. He was a financial advisor. I think we would have run him off if she hadn't told us her wishes. I'm almost sure we would have. We didn't want a civilian running this place. She stayed in Mobile. She was here before the war and stayed right on through.

She was going to build a new hospital and that's what she did. To show you what kind of a person she was: my grandmother was a diabetic and had to have her leg amputated from gangrene, quite a common thing in those days, still is. But there were a hell of a lot more then at the old hospital. They had just added a new wing of ten or 12 beds and Poppa and his brother wanted to dedicate one of the rooms: furnish one of the new rooms and dedicate it, and put the bronze plaque on the door. They spelled the damn name wrong. They spelled it R-U-M-P-A-N-O-U instead of O-S. I called White-Spunner's attention to it and she said it's going to have to stay that way, because I'll be damned if I'm going to buy a new plaque. She said we were going to be in the new hospital before long anyhow. She said it like it was.

That thing stayed there. She didn't make a change. I wouldn't dare ask her to do so. She was good. Heck I had pneumonia one time and she didn't have a bed anywhere. She put a bed up in her office for me. And Warren from X-ray, a black man that really ran the X-ray department down there, had pleural effusion. I'm sure it was TB. There weren't admitting blacks then. She didn't . . . White-Spunner didn't do it, but she knew we did. She had Ms. Baumgardner let us have a bed and we set it up down in the onion bin at the old Mobile Infirmary. Put this black guy down there that worked for the hospital. We had to tap his chest every two or three days to keep him alive. He's still living. Baumgardner gave us the bed.

We would get these Creoles, the Rivers and all, from up at Citronelle and everything. We couldn't admit them, but we'd go downstairs and operate on them. I think they had an aneurysm, one of them, back in the popliteal area. I fixed an aneurysm on one and we didn't have an outpatient room or an emergency room and if anybody came in we'd have to take them up to the operating room. I don't know what room I did it in. It was in some room downstairs. He had refused to go to the City. Nobody would and I couldn't admit him to Mobile or Providence. The hospital just looked the other way.

I think after the war was one of my best times because I had a lot to do—stuff that was just lying around here that nobody was doing. I did all kinds of stomach cases: bypassing ulcers instead of doing the big resections. Those first few years after the war were fun. Looking back the only thing I really like to look at is that I practiced over 50 years and never had a suit. I never even had a threat of one. Talking, being frank with patients got me away from that. Talking to them. If it was something I didn't think I could do I would find them somebody better. Follow up on everything.

CHAPTER 7

Harry Newell Webster, Jr., MD (1915–2006)

Physician

University of Alabama 1937

Jefferson Medical College, Philadelphia 1941

Opened Mobile practice 1941

Interviewed 2001 at 86 years old

I rode the ambulance and I was an intern. That's how I came here. I went to school in Philadelphia and I was so tired of snow and ice and Yankees until I wanted to come home. I picked out a place that was closest to my home, which was Evergreen, Alabama, for my internship. Foster was an ambulance driver. He was one of the younger ones and he didn't stay there as long as the others before. There were two that stayed there for years and years and years. I can only remember the name of one of them by his nickname, which was Wimpy. The other one, his name will come back to me. But those two were there and they had a little sleeping room in the back and they stayed on 24 hours a day for the time that they were there and then the other came and took over and they stayed through a 24-hour shift. At City Hospital.

I was born on September 15, 1915, in Flomaton, Alabama. My father was an employee of the American Telephone and Telegraph Company; spent his whole life at that. I was reared in Evergreen, Alabama. Went to school there until I left to go to school at the University of Alabama to go to premed and then I got a BS and I went into the medical school.

To become a doctor, my whole idea I think, I never had any other idea about it and I expect I had lots of reasons, because my favorite aunt was a registered nurse. I'm sure that she had a lot to do with stimulating me in wanting to go into medicine. I got a lot of advice about it, about how to be a doctor. She was more interested that I not mistreat nurses. If you're going to be a doctor, don't you dare mistreat the nurses. So, I learned my dos and don'ts about relationships between doctors and nurses from my aunt. Her name was Ola Adela Cochran. She was familiarly known all her life as Della, because of Adela. She was mother's oldest sister. She was working all over the place. She was a shaker and mover.

She went off for her original training at the University of Missouri and got her advanced degree. In those days that was unusual. She wound up owning and operating a hospital. She was a mover. As a nephew and because I was interested, I was always invited to be there. And so I was there when they actually opened up the hospital and I got to see the nurses and doctors. So it was a natural thing for me to want to get into medicine. I went to the University of Alabama School of Medicine.

Two-year program because that's all there was in Alabama at that time. All students had to be transferred out to junior status to the other medical schools, to the other teaching universities. Attrition rate in those days for medical students was high. We didn't have very much. If you wanted to go to medical school you'd say here I am and here's my tuition. You're in. Sure, I'll flunk you out in the first three months and you'll go on home. That's the way they weeded them out in those days. It was not unusual to see fellows that you lived with just pack their bags and go home, just scared to death.

I graduated from medical school in 1941, and I graduated from Alabama in 1937, and I must have gone in 1932. I was there for six years. I stayed there for a four-year undergraduate term where I got my BA degree and did two years in medicine, so I was there for a total of six years, in Tuscaloosa. Then at that time there was a fight to get the favorite place that you wanted.

There were not many places open for a junior admission, you see, so there was always a bridge you had to cross to be able to go to the school you wanted to go to. Of course, I had two schools in mind at that time. One of them was Tulane and the other was Jefferson College in Philadelphia. I knew Tulane because of its proximity and I knew Jefferson was a good college because several of my good friends who were in classes ahead of me had fought one another tooth and nail to be sure they got in and they did. So I had friends who were already up there so I wanted to go. I went. I was fortunate enough that they selected me. Not before they gave me heart failure because they waited so long to do it! They didn't answer and didn't answer and here I sit. Everybody else is getting accepted in school here and school there.

The dean of the two-year school at Alabama had the responsibility to get everybody transferred out. He would call me every three or four days and say Mr. Webster have you sent your money in? He had already gotten me a place in South Carolina where I didn't want to go. I didn't want to tell him that I didn't want to go to South Carolina. He said, have you sent your money, and I'd say, no sir, I'm waiting to hear from Jefferson. I'd signed up for Jefferson. That's how I got off to Pennsylvania to go to school.

My family was very supportive. My mother, bless her heart, she was in my corner 100 percent of the time, all of the time. Without her support I couldn't have done it. My father felt like I was already a college graduate and I ought to go out and go get a job and that kind of stuff. I sort of felt that way. I was getting to be a pretty good size boy and I'd come home from school and seen all of my friends that I graduated from high school with, married and got dogs and children and here I am with books under my arm going to school, still a schoolboy.

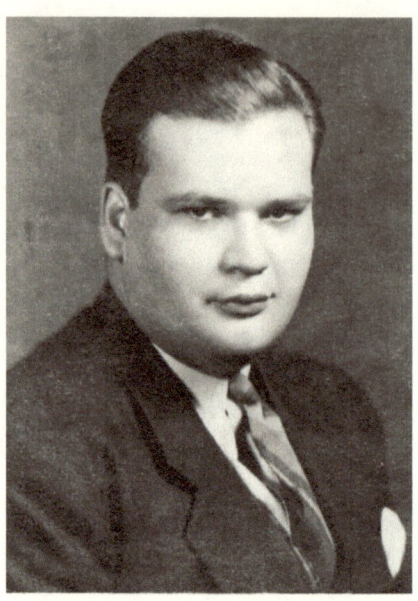

Dr. Harry N. Webster, Jr. (1942). He opened his Mobile, Alabama, practice in 1941. Dr. Webster planned from the outset to become a general practitioner.

From Tuscaloosa, Goodman, my real good friend, Leo M. Goodman who finally wound up with a successful internship out in Sacramento, California, was already in Philadelphia. The other fellow from Alabama was Clement Lightcap, he was in my class at the University of Alabama but he was Phi Chi and I was a Phi Beta Pi and never the twain shall meet. So, I went to Philadelphia several weeks early looking for some job to sort of curtail the expenses. This was Depression years and there wasn't much money and you could get a pretty good meal for 35 cents. But you needed a place to sleep and I didn't have rent to pay. At that time I was able to be a lab technician, so I went to Blair Hospital close to the university trying to find a spot as a night technician so I could work at night and go to school in the daytime. But things were so tough then and nobody wanted to hire anybody and any job that there was around, everybody had some local person that they wanted. So I didn't get a job there.

But I got a job on a truck that was spreading concrete. All those old homes, row homes, were heated by coal and they had a coal bin—the basement was a coal bin. They had just gone over to oil. Now instead of having them a bin down there they had a big tank-like job with oil in it.

Then they all of a sudden had a big room down there that they wanted to fix, so what we were doing was backing in this truck loaded with concrete, putting it in the coal chute, going down there. And I was down in the bottom moving concrete around to put a floor in! That's the work I did while I was waiting for school to open.

When school opened, Clement Lightcap was there to register and of course we got together and started to talk and we decided we would be better off if we went together and got an efficiency apartment, which I had already found. We did that and we stayed in that efficiency apartment for the two years we were there. To make the story even better, after he went on in the Army, I didn't get in the Army. I was drafted into being the local physician at Alabama Dry Dock and Shipbuilding. They had to have somebody over there at that time to run the emergency, the first aid, take care of injuries, so I was there. That kept me from being taken into the service, but Clem went on into the service.

In Philadelphia I had the last two years of medical school. There I got into the clinical work. The University of Alabama had done all the scientific, basic work: histology, anatomy, chemistry, physiology, all the basics were ground into us. We had a pretty good basic training because they were having to prepare us to be transferred. They didn't want to send a clunker to one of those schools, because then they couldn't transfer anybody else up there. They didn't send out the clunkers. You didn't pass to get by, you went home. I was ready to go into the advanced training. I still had to do some anatomy. I remember I had to take a course in cross-sectional anatomy, which I hadn't had. But, with the basics that I had, I had no real problem on any of it. The big problem for me was to maintain my grade average and transfer out to wherever I wanted to for an internship. You know I didn't want to be the last man in the class either, so I worked my tuchus off.

I didn't know what I was going to do until I came here. I knew what I wanted to do when I came out: I wanted to treat the skin and its contents. I was going to be a general practitioner and that's what I wanted to do. And that's sort of the reason I came here. At that time, Mobile was run by people who had those characteristics. Surgery was done by the general practitioners; obstetrics was done by the general practitioners. There wasn't hardly anybody who had a clear practice, maybe there were two or three. I can remember an ear, eye, nose, and throat man who didn't do anything but that. And I think there was a proctologist, who didn't do anything but that. A radiologist, pathologist, and then everybody else did everything. The surgeons delivered babies and, you know, treated colds and coughs, sprains and fractures.

That was it: if you were in medicine that was it. Nobody asked me what I wanted to be. They said you're on duty and right now you've got to take care of those wards over there. So I was assigned to a couple of wards over there at the City Hospital. And then I rotated through that. Another thing I had to do: I had to attend all of the pathological studies. I had to do all the autopsies and that sort of thing. So I got a lot of things to do. Dr. Wert came and took over from me. I was acting pathologist for the City Hospital. The pathologist there had moved on to other fields and they didn't have anybody. I was serving as pathologist for them when Wert came. So when he came out I greeted him with joy and relief. We've been friends for years.

During that time, Tommy Boudreaux, who is the father of the Tommy Boudreaux who is over at the Mobile Infirmary, was a trained urologist. Then I began to work with him and he taught me how to use the cystoscope and do all the things and [I] became more and more interested in that. After about six or seven years of general practice, one day decided that I really wanted to be a urologist. So then I was a urologist. I sent out notices to all my patients and let them know. Then I starved for about six months and then it picked up.

Board certification was there. Board certification at the time when I started in was largely the amount of applying for a certificate and getting it. It became much more difficult. Board certification became a way of detecting two things: it ensured that everybody had a good education that went into it; it also protected the territory from interlopers, which had been people who came in like I did. Just open the door and say here I am, I'm a urologist, don't you forget it. You know?

But, that would not have worked, wouldn't have worked for me if I had wanted to go to New Orleans. But it worked for me here because I had then established a presence with the community. They knew who I was and what I was and whether I was able to do that. Of course if I hadn't done with Boudreaux and then I took over the practice of a noted urologist who decided he wanted to be an anesthesiologist. That was Dr. Claude Mastin Cleveland. He had them lined up doing nothing but anesthesia for all the hospitals in town. When he started doing that he couldn't take care of his urology anymore, so I filled out whatever year he had left. It wasn't much because he had started doing more anesthesia.

I was working down at the docks: Alabama Dry Dock and Shipbuilding Company, which is right across the river where they build ships. And they, at the time I was over there, were building Liberty ships. They were docking one of them there every five or six weeks. Now you would have called it occupational medicine. You didn't call it that then. You could call it whatever you wanted to, nobody gave it a name because it wasn't that much and if you said you were a specialist in occupational medicine, nobody would have known what you were talking about.

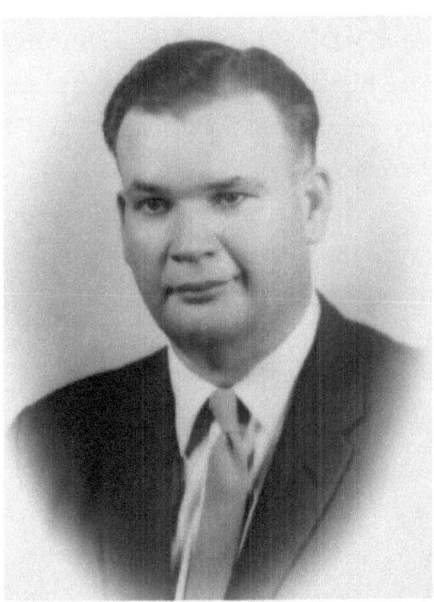

Dr. Webster started working at ADDSCO in 1944 (undated photo)

I was at the City Hospital even when I did that. I stayed at City Hospital. City Hospital was a charity hospital. There wasn't anybody making any money up there, but there were people over there who were sick and needed to be taken care of. I had been there for years and I never quit. I stayed right there and I did free care as long as I could stay in it. I really did two things. I went over and I would go and be at the place and I would be on call over there all of the time. I had to get a night crew at the docks. We had a little hospital over there and I had about 30 patients over there at the time. It was a pretty good size when they were building as many ships as they built over there. It was a big business.

As a matter of fact, by the time I had been at the docks about six or eight months and the state Public Health Service came to review over there and said you've got to have help boy. I said I sure do, so they sent me some help. I got three recruits that they got from New York where they take these doctors up there and put them in uniform for the United States Department of Public Health Service. Then they would send them wherever they wanted to go. They'd do that rather than to be shipped over to get shot at. So suddenly I had help.

At the time I went to ADDSCO (Alabama Dry Dock and Shipbuilding Company), I had carte blanche as to organizing. I no longer had a boss. I answered to nobody except the president of ADDSCO. And so I had a hospital down there with eight beds and four operating rooms. I stayed busy 24 hours a day, taking care of the needs of all the people over there: at that time there were about 25 people there so certainly I had a chance to staff it as I saw fit. So I started out knowing that I had to recruit and I wanted the best, so I raised the pay. I paid more than anybody else in town. I don't remember how much it was but I got a lot of criticism from the hospital. I wanted the best—they had to act on their own a lot of times. I didn't have time to train everybody so I had to hire the best I could and with a carte blanche I could do that. So I'm going to take credit for the first place that medicine ever got benefits for nurses.

Hospitals had nurse trainees because it was cheaper, cheap labor. They also had interns. My salary as an intern was five dollars a month. I lived in the hospital. The nurses lived in the hospital. The food was free: you got food, lodging, and five dollars a month. The nuns ran it and if the nuns liked you they sent you five dollars every Sunday and a bottle of whiskey. You couldn't ever tell when you were going to get that. That was because you got something from the nuns. I would go back to my bed, which was on the other side of the library, the interns' quarters, a series of rooms with bunk beds in them. In my bed, I would have my whiskey, and I got a lot of thinking done. That was at City Hospital and I stayed there until I left to go practice with Joe Little.

Some of the other physicians at that time were Dr. Boudreaux; Doring was one of the eyes, ear, nose, and throat men: he was an interesting character. He was way ahead of the game when he came and he was just as busy as he could be. He didn't associate much with anybody else because he didn't need to go to the hospital. He did all his work in his office. I got to know him some and I enjoyed him. Being in his company was—it was amusing to deal with someone that was so far outside of my usual run of acquaintances. But he was one that the other eye, ear, nose, and throat men would hope would come by when he got to be 85 years old.

Seagrest was an internist. Acker was a longtime chief of surgery at the City Hospital. He was a very old man the first time I ever saw him. I don't know how old he was but he seemed old to me. He was from the old, old school and he believed in . . . only used iodine and no narcotics at all. Had a hard time giving them to his patients who were in pain. Thought that was the wrong thing to do. But I just remember that.

Heiter was my good friend and I got tied up a good many years as a surgical assistant and learned a lot about surgery from him. You learned in those days, even assistants did. Sooner or later, as time went on, he began to let me do more and more of the surgery because I was, to tell you the truth, more adept at it than he was.

The Donalds came late. I knew the Donalds from the time they went into school, the older boy. He went to Philadelphia the year before I did. He went to the University of Pennsylvania. I only knew that he was there because I ran into him at one of the hospitals where I tried to go get a job; he already had the job, so I didn't get it! That was the older one and then after the war he came here and of course by that time I had already well established in practice and could give him a good start.

When the physicians experienced by the war began to return to town, they brought some new techniques back and anybody who came in with something new, I picked their brains just as quick as I could because that's the way I wanted to learn. I've always learned by picking other people's brains. That's the way you do it, you know. Somebody knows it better than you, shut your mouth and go over there and watch them do it and if you can get your hand in the blood too you can learn something.

There are other ways that things come, new things. When some fellows learn something new, he wants to get full; he wanted everybody to hear that he could. So he gets on his typewriter and types a paper, tells what he is doing. And before long everybody is talking about it you know, and they type down the same notes that he had and see how he did off from what the usual practice was and whether that was an improvement. So, I watched a lot of things, including stage two prostatectomy, stage one prostatectomy, the perineal prostatectomy, the transurethral resection of the prostate. All the rest came along as I came along and we had to learn each one of those things as another jump.

Continuous learning: that's something that I give great credit to Dr. Earl Wert. Earl came and took over from there. I'll tell you, he took my place as the pathologist at City Hospital and pretty soon he was also pathologist for Mobile Infirmary. Both of them. But early on we had the best group of physicians who were meeting together with some regularity to discuss medicine at that place. So he was ideal for that. He began to lead those discussions . . . it was before the tissue committee came along. The tissue committee came later.

Pathology conferences is what you call them. And Earl would seek out all the pathological specimens, teaching things, and once a week we met in the library at the City Hospital, that was the first clinical teaching that was ever done in Mobile on any kind of regular basis and it was wonderful. It was real interesting to listen to everybody's take on whatever Earl was presenting. He was a good pathologist and is a good teacher, a very intelligent man. He did a great job of that I want to say. I remember that after it had been going on a short time, something really unusual happened. We all got together and tried to reward him and so we gave him a gold watch. I haven't thought about it in years. Anyway, he was raising everybody's awareness of the value of continuing medical education and that was the first anything like an active lecture that came here and he did it for a long time.

He and one of the Donalds broke up ghost surgery. Oh yeah. Ghost surgery was the fact that internists would tell a patient that he would be operated on, and would go out and pick out a surgeon and say I want you to come help me do this. So the surgeon would go do it for a 15-dollar assistant's fee. He would operate for this doctor who couldn't tie his shoelace. Seriously. That was not unusual, that was sort of standard. A doctor who could get somebody else to come do his surgery wouldn't send the patient on referral to Donald, who didn't do anything but surgery. That was his right; he wasn't going to get anything as long as people were doing surgery for 15 dollars for the fellows who had the patients.

Now the surgeons, the fellow who did that, couldn't keep himself alive doing surgery because he was not—nobody is going to refer him to anything except when he got that. And of course what Donald was hoping was by word of mouth, sooner or later, the public began to know that you were a competent surgeon and you began to get public referrals. There are two kinds of referrals: a public referral and a physician referral. And to get a physician referral when everybody is doing everything is pretty damn hard. So that's that. I have to say that Donald was adamant about it and he broke it up.

He wouldn't do it and when somebody else did it, I suspect that he clinched it. You know, "You're not going to get by with this, this is unprofessional," and whatever and the first thing you know doctors who were my friends began to quit doing ghost surgeries. It was also when things began to pick up. I remember when I was damn glad to get a ten-dollar surgeon fee. Hell, yes. I pay a lot more taxes now than I made. I paid more taxes in six months than I made in six years before. Times were tough and I can remember when I made twenty thousand dollars one year and that was just wonderful. I made twenty thousand dollars in a year!

When I started into practice, in the Medical Society, a membership automatically got you into all the hospitals. You said, here am I, and they said, we're glad to have you. Except that I had an interesting go with Providence Hospital: I had been in private practice only a short time when all of the sudden I had a call from one of the sisters out there, the head sister, and she wanted to know why I had admitted a patient out there. She said well, you're not a member of the staff. I said Sister, I guess I'm not, but I've been working out there for five years. So that was sort of the end of that. I think I must have gotten admitted to the staff right then! That's the only place I ever had a question from the hospital. You just go down and work in their hospital.

I think the Mobile Infirmary must have had, when I started, they must have had one hundred beds or so. It was really a small hospital. It was at that time the only hospital not under the control of the Catholic Church. That's what made the difference. That's why it was there. The local people had wanted a hospital that was not sect-based. So what they did was they said this is going to be something other than that. So all the other churches in town and got behind this idea and they made up a pot and started up a hospital, which was the Mobile Infirmary.

Ms. White-Spunner was here running the hospital when I came. A lovely lady and one of my very favorite people in the all the world. Katherine White-Spunner was not a beauty. But Katherine White-Spunner was a forceful, caring, compassionate person. She was [a] big woman. I often think that she and Eleanor Roosevelt were very similar in size, shape, and presence. Do you know about Eleanor Roosevelt? Well, I want to tell you that she could pass paths with Eleanor and hold her end up. She could control physicians by stomping her foot!

Stomp {her} foot on the floor, damn! When she said that, nobody wanted to hear the next part of it. Nobody ever pushed her any further than that! She would stomp her foot and walk off and there you were standing there with your mouth hanging open. She knew when you had transgressed and she knew why and she knew what to do. She had enough presence so that she was able to control a cantankerous bunch of doctors. She was the boss.

The way she did it was that she was liked. As I say, she was caring and compassionate and for instance, my mother got sick and there wasn't a hospital bed over there, she made up her bed and put my mother in it and she went out and stayed with her family so my mother would have a place to be in the hospital. This is the kind of person she was.

She stayed there until the hospital was rebuilt out on the golf course and then she began to need help because it began to be a big thing. It had 175 beds and it was growing. So she got a young man for an assistant and it didn't take him long for the doctors to run him off. Oh hell no, they were used to Ms. White-Spunner. They didn't want no little squirt coming in telling us what to do. He didn't have a chance, but they really needed somebody to help with the financials of purchasing and all that sort of thing. That's when Pete Bramlett came in. Pete Bramlett worked for the bank and had just come back from the Navy. And there was a gentleman down there who was running the bank who was a great friend of the hospital and always was. He sent Pete out when this other man left.

Pete came and he found his place in life. As soon as he got there, he began to learn and he didn't begin by making anybody angry. He didn't try to supplant Ms. White-Spunner. He never pushed himself forward at all. Then he went to all of the educational opportunities to learn how to be a hospital administrator. The first thing you know he was certified as a hospital administrator. I was proud of him, too. Then, when Ms. White-Spunner finally did retire, he took over the job.

In my office I did not have a separated waiting room. But I didn't have a place for them to sit together. My office had a big hall that led off from the entrance room, which was the waiting room, and my personal business office was up there. My offices were in the back. I had an office, equipment room, an X-ray room. I did my own cystoscopy and X-ray work back there at that time because it was necessary. Patients at that time were not covered with insurance. So I got an X-ray machine so I could make my own X-rays. Nobody needs to do that now. I had all of that back there. But in this hallway I had chairs and that's where my colored patients sat. I don't remember ever telling one of them to sit there, but that's where they knew to sit.

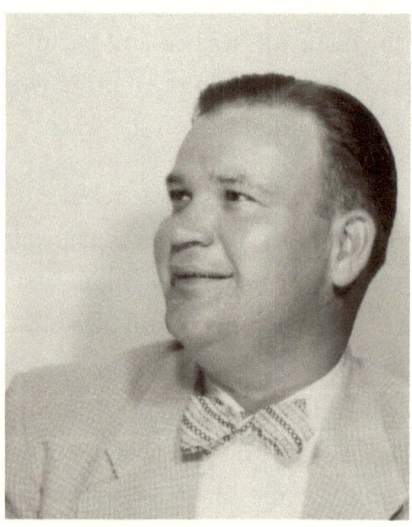

Dr. Harry Newell Webster, Jr. (1950)

It didn't make any difference. They were taken as quickly as anybody else and they got the same treatment as anybody else. I told the colored patients, all of them that I had, I enjoyed having them. I wasn't trying to run them off. But, I didn't want them in our hospital. I didn't want the hospital . . . the Mobile Infirmary was all white. The City Hospital was accepting blacks, so was the Providence. Well at that time, it was still lily-white.

I really kind of wanted it that way because I had so much trouble with substandard help, not from all of them, but with some of the blacks. They soon began to tell everybody with the same breath, "but that's wrong." But that's what you do. And so I really felt that it was worth staying lily-white and I tried to keep it that way as long as I could. But there came a time when anybody had to know that there had to be a change, including an old country boy like me raised up there in swamps of Conecuh. Exceptions provided. There was nothing to be ashamed of. They had to be in the room next door. You know, you don't put them in a separate place or anything. It was only right, but it was a change and one that was hard to come by when you have a lifetime of apartheid. It didn't start in South Africa. They didn't start that. They just sort of stayed in their place. I stayed in mine too. I didn't go. We were separate. The law said equal was separate. But of course it never was. It was awful hard to get equality. Everything that has equality has gotten a rise and fall on either side.

Getting into the Medical Society was difficult. It was a difficulty for me because I came here at a time when all of the physicians had been rooted out and sent to the service. They cleaned the place out. Since I didn't go and hadn't been here before and I'd never been a member of the society, the elder of the group said we're not going to take any more members in until these boys get back. You go ahead and do anything you want to do, but you can't be a member of the society.

Now that stayed on for about two years, I think, and then they responded and let me in, I don't know why. But it didn't bother me one way or the other, because it didn't mean anything because it didn't keep us from being a member of the hospital and practicing anywhere I wanted to. I was not accepted the first time I applied. It was just the fellows who was left, and largely they were led by, I'm trying to remember whose nose was out of joint over the competition. A lot of these doctors went together and made it a mission to grab all of the practices for themselves, the practices that were left high. They usually bought them or . . . I know that one of my friends was a general surgeon, he went off. He sold his rights to his practice to a local physician, who then went out and hired physicians from somewhere else and brought them in. This made these people very angry: that here is a new doctor coming in to take over this practice, that had never been here before.

That was a problem that was not a clear-cut problem. But the real problem gradually did surface. There are always two sides to every pancake. I don't recall that there was any great day of reckoning, you might say, that it was clear today and it wasn't clear yesterday. This is something that gradually improved as they began accepting. Places who had a doctor, didn't want another one there. Doctors didn't want another doctor coming in their area. It's my business right now. You're my competition. Right now I've got it and you come in here and you can do it a little better and smile a little prettier and a little sooner, and you're going to have some of my business and my pocketbook is going to get lighter. And so you and I are going to get clear. There were doctors and that was the days before when a lump of sugar paid the bill and then everybody started laughing all the way to the bank.

Insurance came in. Some of those plants had health care schemes and they were insured to the extent that they paid the doctor bills. At the time I came here those plants were paying for all of the injuries and all of the occupational medicine and there were doctors here who did nothing else but occupational medicine. They say they were in occupational medicine; they say they were surgeons. They had a contract with International Paper, with the oil company, all those people had special doctors. They sent all of their patients there and they were there to do it. When I went into practice, I went into practice with the doctor who had the shipyard. He was the doctor for the shipyard; his name was Joe Little.

He was a cutter! He was my good friend back then because he knew a ton of women. He and I were always friends and I went down and took a job with him, a paid job, six hundred dollars a month. My God, what money I was making. I went to his office and I bandaged and sewed up cuts and did all that kind of stuff and saw to the patients we had in the hospital and I went out and fixed them up. But in about six months from the time that I started, he closed his office because he went to the Army. Now when he went into the Army, he told me to go on over and start doing the work at the shipyard. I did and I enjoyed doing it. I was challenged from it and did it until I had the chance to get loose from it. I got a chance to get loose from it when a group of surgeons that worked through the United States Department of Public Health Service had been England for the GIs. They came back over and they needed a place so they said we can put those in there.

I said come on. So pretty soon they were in there and I got to go out and find me an office. I was in private general practice then until I retired from that and went over to go to work in the hospital, Mobile Infirmary. I was the vice president in charge of medical affairs at Mobile Infirmary for ten years. I went in to see Pete Bramlett and told him that I was getting ready to retire and I had always intended to retire when I was 60. I knew that sooner or later my abilities would suffer because of my advanced age. I've seen it happen before. I would have to go tell Dr. X not to go in the operating room. There ain't no sense. I did that several times and I didn't want anybody to ever have to do that to me.

I had already made arrangements and put a few bucks aside. When I was 60 years old, I told him that I was going to stop general practicing. During that time, I had been stuck in the hospital trying to getting a quality control system set up. They wanted me to come over there and I did. What I took on as a part-time job, became a full-time job. A few years got to be ten before too long and I was 70 and I quit.

The difference between the Providence and the Infirmary at that time was only that some things were taken care of better at one hospital and other things were taken care of better at the other hospital. Early on we had better obstetrical situation over at Providence than at Mobile. When one would get better at something, it made the other come up to it, so it didn't stay that way for long. But you always have some differences and they were always trying to maintain premier status. There were some doctors who would not go to Providence because they did not want to practice at Providence because of the church. That was a problem. Another thing if you wanted to do an operation that wound up with sterility you had a problem with the Catholic Church. So you couldn't do very much that was obstetrical or gynecological, particularly when you were going to do a hysterectomy or tie the tubes. You could not do that at Providence. If a woman needed her tubes tied, she had to go to the Infirmary for it.

Nobody did abortions, nobody knew about it when an abortion was done. There was a doctor downtown who did abortions. I saw the man one time. It—the results—it was a horror and I had to clean up his messes because . . . it was a bad, bad disease, we didn't have much to do with it. Lots of girls died from septic abortions. They could go to New Orleans, have the abortion, and get septic by the time they got back here. Oh yeah, it was terrible. Abortion was unregulated, against the law, and dangerous and I'm sure that there were abortions done that I didn't know anything about because it could be done surreptitiously. But I didn't know of many and the doctor didn't want anybody to know about it because he did not want the reputation. It was against the law—you could spend some time in jail for that.

The Allen Memorial was built as a Zion for unwed Catholic mothers. That's what it started out. They could go over there if they got pregnant and spend their time, that's where they had their baby and the baby was adopted. They could go over there until they got over their pregnancy, disappear from their family. The family said she's off taking a beauty course. They didn't want to say that she's waiting to have a baby. It was not a happy situation, it's not happy now; truthfully it is more unhappy than it is happy, but the bonus of having it done is it's not too bad. But beyond the tale, which is most of us can't stand it. I don't want to be the one to do abortions, but I don't want to have to put up with it either. I've got other things I want to do.

When I was practicing, those patients with depression or psychiatric issues, those that could be taken care of, got sedation. It was a challenge if they were young. The person who had real psychological problems, particularly those that had any manic manifestations, wound up in jail. We soon came to understand that really wasn't the right place for them so we fixed up a psychiatric ward so the jail wouldn't have to have them anymore. We got that because the sheriff said that I ain't gonna have that anymore. He wanted to be rid of us.

Alcoholics and addicts: we avoided them as much as possible. Drug addicts drove me crazy because they'd call me all hours of the night for something to get them out of trouble; it's hard to get a hold of and it's hard to carry on. I had some that wanted me to give them some narcotics. They tried every way they could. Thank goodness I don't get that kind of call anymore. They never were welcome. People with narcotics problems need help and even now I'm not sure they get the kind of help they should have. We didn't have any decent way of taking care of alcoholics. The first real care they got was Alcoholics Anonymous. They do some great work. It's a way to get people dry and a lot of them stay dry. I would respond to AA calls whenever I could. I wanted to do whatever I could do. As time went on, I believe there was better help for them; certainly, the recognition that alcoholism is a disease and not a matter of morality helped.

I got married August 1942. I got my internship and the war had come on and I took this job over at the shipyard where they were building ships for the war. My job was such that they wouldn't take me into the Army or Navy. So I had to stay with that. I met this nice young lady who I fell in love with and stayed in love for, do the math, '42 to now. She was from Mobile. She had a place as a nurse at City Hospital in private practice. I got to courting her and we got married and been married ever since.

CHAPTER 8

Samuel Eichold, MD (1916–2006)

Internist

Tulane University 1936

Tulane University Medical School 1940

Opened Mobile practice 1945

Interviewed on 4/13/00 at 84 years old

I was born here in 1916, May 27. Let me say to you, the reason I went to medical school was because I wanted to be a physician. In the first grade, I sat at the desk and the teacher passed around a little paper that we had—the *Public School Courier*—and said what do you want to be when you're grown? And I said, "I want to be a doctor. I do not want to be a surgeon. I want to be a diagnostician." And the teacher couldn't spell diagnostician! So that's when I made it clear what I wanted to do and I never deviated from that one minute. I had an uncle who was a physician. And I don't remember thinking I'd rather do anything else.

Then I was blessed to be with a bunch of doctors who were willing to let a kid watch them. Dr. O'Gwynn was an otolaryngologist. I mean I would hold down the tongue while he would do tonsillectomies in the office. I was maybe ten years old, twelve years old. Those days it was so easy to practice medicine without a license.

Dr. Doehring used to say, now Sam let's not argue about when I want the tongue blade, you give it to me and I'll take over. I was standing on a little running board by the chair. He did surgery in the old O'Gwynn Building on Conception and Conti Street. There was a museum in that building, on the second floor where the reception room was. The offices were on the second and third floors. Dr. O'Gwynn and Dr. McGehee, they encouraged me to be a doctor; that's why I studied medicine. Most don't have that opportunity.

For years I took care of Dr. McGehee. Tiny McGehee, P. D. McGehee. Dr. McGehee, as my mother described: "like Jesus." He was just a marvelous guy. Day and night he was on call and he never, never questioned if they needed a doctor. He was there. He would go in the house and be just as friendly as I would be with you if I had walked in the house with you. And he'd come out and say I like to wring her damn neck! He was just contained, his passion—never showed it. Very amazing person. He made house calls. He'd come by and pick me up at 6:30 in the morning and take me over to the hospital for surgery and then make rounds, then leave the office about 6:30 p.m. or 7:00 to make the hospital calls; house calls until 9:30 p.m.. He was in the office every day. Ms. Forbes was his nurse through all this. Always accused him of having an affair with his nurse, but she was just a devoted, loving, attentive person and [had] a very interesting manner. Her devotion was great. Dr. McGehee and Dr. E. J. Beck were associates, not partners. They worked together; they were independent, but associated, with shared responsibilities. They didn't need a formal agreement.

I was 15. I was driving the car. He had a big Cadillac and had to have hydraulic brakes installed because I was so short and to effectively manage it we needed that. I just took care of him, in the sense of making rounds, carrying the bag, going from room to room in the hospital. I remember seeing cases of pellagra they showed me. We didn't see it often, and if they pointed it out to you in the beginning, you didn't forget. McGehee was in the Van Antwerp Building, on the fifth floor. He had his office downtown, but he'd treat anybody, anywhere.

He saw a total cross section in the office, I remember that. Calls he made during the day and Mrs. Forbes, she made out bills in the afternoon. He was just furious if you called in another doctor. My dad, I never will forget, had a hernia and I decided Dr. Herbert Cole should do the surgery and Dr. McGehee would assist. Dr. McGehee was just furious about the disloyalty. Dr. McGehee would make house calls. He was a source of great relief in the community. For example, some of the female population would need an emotional outlet. They would tell Dr. McGehee, I just don't feel good, he'd come by and say your blood pressure is awful low, honey, you just stay in bed now for a few days. But every day, two times a day, for years he saw patients. In those days house calls were three dollars. We had no antibiotics. We had no therapeutic modalities. The medicines we used were Prontosil—a red liquid for infections—and that was the only thing we had. This was pre–sulfa drugs, maybe 1935–1936. Dr. Doehring brought it from Germany. It was a liquid, it was injectable. Later, after World War II we had sulfanilamide, sulfadiazine, and sulfathiazole.

As an undergraduate student I went to Tulane. At the end of my junior year in medical school I got a "condition" in psychology. It turns out I had to pass a conditioning class—make up the exam late that summer in order to enter medical school in the fall; entered medical school in 1936 in Tulane. In Alabama and Mississippi there were only two-year schools. That's why all of us from Alabama went to medical school in New Orleans. Tulane was a four-year school—gave us uninterrupted continuity. There was a flood of application by the New England students to Tulane. They maybe couldn't get into the bigger Ivy League schools. There were a bunch of bright Jews in New England who maybe couldn't get into Harvard, Yale, or the rest of them. Tulane had a quota to fill but they were partial to Southern men.

The only time I ever worked with the dog lab was when, in medical school, a fellow used to sharpen our knives in anatomy. A dark-complected man, Zeno was his name and he worked with the dogs. His job was to debark the dogs because the neighbors in that area, in the big affluent subdivision around Tulane, were disturbed. So they wanted to get rid of the dogs. Instead of that we just cut their vocal cords; the vocal cords on dogs. They were perfectly healthy dogs. It was Zeno's job, but he let me do it. I was always looking for a new experience.

Dr. Alton Ochsner was the chairman of the department of surgery. He was a real taskmaster. My father, who owned a surgical supply company, had sent me some information about a Miller-Abbot tube. I mentioned what I had learned about it slightly in a discussion with Dr. Ochsner. He remembered me after that. My friend Hamm Newman, a New Orleans boy, had just started on his surgical rotation about one month. Dr. Ochsner started his rounds about 6 a.m. That meant we had to be up and going by 5 a.m. to be prepared for Ochsner. A patient was in distress and Dr. Ochsner asked the nurse what she had done. She had called Hamm during the night and he had prescribed over the phone—he had not seen the patient in person. Dr. Ochsner asked him if he had even seen that patient. Ham said, "Yes, sir." Ochsner kept asking him questions and he kept saying, "Yes, sir." He was under such pressure that he didn't answer with the facts, only, "Yes, sir." It sounded like he lied. Ochsner got mad and said, "You're out! And you're"—pointing to me—"going to take his place." It all ended well, and he was a marvelous teacher.

I finished in 1940 and wanted to intern at Touro but didn't have good enough grades. Mine were in the middle of the class and Touro required real top students. I went to Dr. Isadora Cohn, a protégée of Matas, to ask about it. I visited more people and ultimately gained my internship at Touro.

In Mobile, Dr. Lee Roe had started the Tuberculosis Sanitarium. Sol Kahn had the Panama Overall Co.—the first unionized garment plant in Alabama—and supported his replacement by Dr. Sam Romandi, a New England doctor. At that time we weren't integrated. For a long time we had separate colors in different rooms. These patients were long term. It helped everyone to have families, wives and children who came to stay with patients, in a more compatible arrangement. The reasoning was that if the patient and their family were not happy they wouldn't heal nor would they stay. Departure was just as big an issue as healing. We had light-complected people in the same room, dark-complected people in the same room. They were kept segregated. And the federal government mandated integration. And this federal agent said to Dr. Romandi, "You're segregating patients. You don't know what it is to be segregated." Dr. Romandi called him a damn fool and said, "I was born and raised a Jew in the ghetto in New York City! I know what segregation is!" It was all the talk for a while, how Dr. Romandi had told off the federal agent.

It was not that feeling in the South towards the Eastern European, but it was toward Catholic, Protestant, and Jew. In Mobile we were a segregated, stratified society. The Athleston Club was a social club started after the Masonic lodge began on the corner of St. Joseph and Dauphin Streets. So, the Athleston Club was Protestant, some Catholics became members, but it did discriminate against Jews. There were clandestine lodges for the blacks, the Fidelia Club for Jews, and other clubs in town for non-Jews.

In Mobile, the old City Hospital was downtown, in front of the Marine Hospital, which had been the District Tuberculosis Hospital and closed 8/52. Mr. J. L. Bedsole rebuilt the hospital in memory of his sister. The architect they had was as crooked as a ram's horn and ended up in jail for paying under-the-table bids for municipal contracts. Anyway it was an architectural abortion what he did to that building.

So anyway I left Touro in 1941 and went to City Hospital for my residency. I would see more cases in one week in Mobile that I could in a year at Touro. I was a member of the Naval Reserve and had been at City Hospital maybe six or eight weeks, that was all the formal training I had, when I was called to active duty. They felt training was not as important as dedication. Doctors Grady Segrest, H. S. J. Walker, and J. C. O'Gwynn were teachers. When I came back from the service they said you're six months short on training and not eligible for the boards. This was regardless of the work I'd done in the service. I'd have to go do a twelve-month residency somewhere.

I had a wife and one child already! You couldn't get a six-month residency. It made me insecure. I think not having my board certification gave me a complex to make myself more knowledgeable.

They were a bunch of veterans who had a feeling of unity in the community. People like Arthur Wood had been sent off to the service by a group of people: the Purdues—C. C., J. D., and W. W. Purdue—and Oswalt. And they shipped them off to the service—all the doctors that they wanted out of the community were sent into the service so they could stay in the community. The community became loaded with mercenaries I would say. Some of them had bags into which they put their money, under the bed. Oh yeah, everything was cash during WWII.

At that time Dr. G. O. Segrest and Acker controlled the Medical Society of Mobile. He told me that I should vote for Cowden's father as president of the Medical Society. I told him I didn't think I could be supportive of him as the authority. Dr. Segrest told Mrs. Marshall, his nurse, not to send any more patients to me again. No referrals. Ever. That was the politics.

Segrest and Purdue created animosity because of the doctors in the community and they had a position that was secure. They were the ones who picked who went off to the war. They shipped off Dr. Oswalt. They shipped out to the recruiting group for the service those people they wanted to go into the service.

Arthur Wood was a leader of the insurgents, he and Bill Sellers. I was overseas and there was one Mobile leader who delegated which ones went overseas and which ones stayed. When the war was over the returning vets began to outnumber the old-timers. To become eligible for admission to the Medical Society everyone individually had to be voted in. Acker would not allow anyone to join—he blackballed each applicant during the vote. Wood said no one is going to join until this gets settled. He was going to hold you *all* back until we get this matter resolved. That was who was going to run the show. But it was not going to be dominated by P. M. J. Acker or Segrest. Acker's got to step down.

Old Dr. Acker had been chairman of the surgical team and ran it with an iron fist. Dr. Segrest was chair of medicine. When I came back in Acker said I couldn't vote because I'm not a member of the staff that has a voting privilege until you serve three years. He denied the privilege to vote! I think he held power as long as he could. He was on the faculty of the old medical college and it closed in 1916. Acker would be in the operating room in his hunting boots. That's true, that's not a story. They even had a sister (DOC [Daughters of Charity]) in there just to wipe the perspiration from his brow. Acker used to say, "Don't wipe, just pat." In those days after they slipped we would push up the glasses on the bridge of his nose. I can see them now putting Dr. Acker's glasses up.

The Daughters of Charity (DOC) were at City Hospital, later Mobile General and finally USA Medical Center. The Sisters of Mercy (SOM) came in to run Blessed Martin de Porres Hospital. I used to say, "Here's how you can tell the two apart: if a piece of paper is on the floor, the DOC sister will call someone in to pick it up; the SOM will pick it up herself."

Before I went overseas I went to see friends and tell them good-bye. That was when Toxy Hayes said to me, "Samuel, you will never be sorry you served." Those were the truest words. There were three Purdues, but J. D., the eldest, he was the boss they accepted, spokesman. A few weeks later a patient of mine came to see me—Dr. Purdue and I shared him—and he said Dr. Purdue said that one day Samuel will be a fine doctor. I never will forget that. It was so nicely said from an older doctor about a younger doctor—finesse. Those are the things you remember.

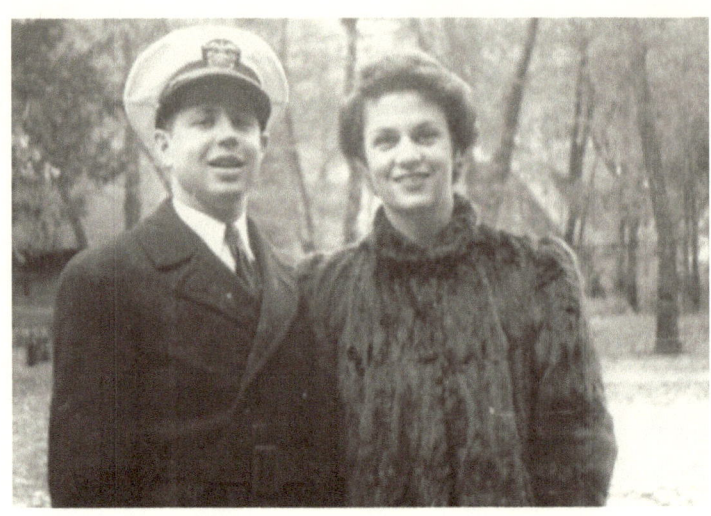

Dr. and Mrs. Sam Eichold (December 1944)

The way I got an office in 1945, office space was zero, nothing was vacant. Bedroom and bath was occupied in Mobile. Nothing was available so I went for a few months to Boston. I left word with Mr. Jimmy Bledsoe of the Van Antwerp Building. He was a close friend of Austill Pharr, president of First National Bank. I prevailed upon them to look for an office for me. So when I came back I had space in the Van Antwerp Building.

In Mobile, on the corner, the policeman was your friend, he'd send patients to you, the elevator man brought you patients, the other doctors in the building referred patients to you. Mobile was packed and jammed. We visited patients two times a day. If they were in the hospital they were real sick and we saw them twice each day. We made three dollars per patient per house call; two dollars per office visit; two dollars for a urine count; two dollars for a blood count.

This was because of the shipbuilding industry in Mobile during World War II. It was a holdover from that. Mobile went through a tremendous growth. And the growth continued after the war was over. Everyone stayed busy. They were grateful to find someone else to share the patient load. We had a steady flow of patients.

Back to the three-room suite in the Van Antwerp Building. It couldn't be segregated because there wasn't enough room to have separate rooms, so we were very discreet. The room was furnished by a fellow by the name of Glen Baylor who was considered a decorator, interior decorator. He had placed a screen or a divider in the room to make it seem more spacious. And it was more or less expected for people to sit where they wanted to sit. And they did. It was never designated or labeled. And somehow or other the screen served the purpose of not being conspicuously segregated. And then there was another area in the hallway. Dr. Walker was across the way from me and he had a large practice with overflow into the chairs in the hallway. And quite often the dark-complected people sat out in the hall out of choice.

We had a dark-complected secretary in the Van Antwerp Building. A patient from Mississippi came in and refused to give his name and address. I went to talk to him and he said he refused to give his name and address to any nigger. I told him that was too bad and good-bye. He walked out. That's just how things were at that time. It was traumatic for her. It was traumatic for me, too!

One time I had a knockdown drag out. I remember saying to Katherine White-Spunner, "Kathy, if a person had an accident on the corner of Ann Street and Springhill Avenue and was brought to the door bleeding (the Mobile Infirmary was down there then—went all the way through to Congress Street), would you admit them?" She said, "No sir, take them to City Hospital." And that was that!

She had been the director of nursing at a Biloxi hospital and she was a member of the White-Spunner family of Mobile. She was the administrator of the Infirmary and Mr. J. L. Bedsole took on the crusade of building the new Mobile Infirmary. He had a marvelous eye for business. The Van Antwerp–Aldridge Surgical Supply Company was started by Mr. J. L. Bedsole and Garrett Aldridge. They brought in Jimmy Bledsole to run it. He became partner and eventually bought it. Mr. J. L. Bedsoe bought it back from him. He had a wholesale drug business and a surgical supply company.

Ed Roberts was president of Waterman Steamship Company. They brought in his brother, Platt, as the architect for the building. It has the same lines, same configuration as the VA hospitals do. They're mostly up north and didn't have to have air conditioning. Miss White-Spunner was convinced the rooms would get a good breeze by being on the hill—she didn't want to get air conditioning. Dr. Beck and Dr. Wood vehemently voiced the need for AC. This was at the time when the physicians were asked for their opinions and preferences. They finally got it. I can remember when it was necessary to have a nurse in the surgery room with a fly-swatter because they got through the screens after the windows had been raised in the heat!

Seventeen years I was in a partnership with Denny Wright. We finally got the money to buy a house and convert it on the corner of Louiselle at Springhill. George Mitchell built his clinic, a women's clinic, across the street from us. We had one reception room and room for three toilet facilities. In that day, you had to have four facilities, one for men, women, black men, and black women. So our office couldn't open because we didn't follow the code, comply with the law. We said we're not going to see any black patients. So that is the story I told. We weren't going to see dark-complected patients which were perfectly legal in 1955. The reception room at Springhill Avenue and Louiselle was one big room and again we used the screen to create a division in the room. People were free to sit where they wanted to. But, on their own accord, they generally sat in groups. But the big lie worked. We stayed open.

Mobile was very fortunate during the segregation years. Joe Langdon, the mayor, who was extremely loyal to all the citizens; Ralph Chandler who published a paper; Bishop Phillips was a dark-complected minister in Mobile; we had Bishop Toolen and several others working together to keep the situation cool. At that time there were two brothers, the Holcombes. One was Bill and one was Bob. The sheriff couldn't succeed himself so one time Bill was the sheriff and the next term Bob was the sheriff. But getting back to the integration era: they absolutely helped Mobile stay peaceful and quiet. If a person wanted to be served at the bus station, they were served.

There was no police problem, we were all very passive and the newspaper was very cooperative. The problem was the actions of the do-gooders who wanted to stir up trouble, create a situation to highlight the discrimination. They chose not to come to Mobile because we didn't respond to them—they couldn't create a stink.

It did affect the delivery of health care. We had a board-certified, dark-complected doctor, Dr. Odom. I knew Dr. Odom was a well-qualified person. He was denied hospital privileges at the Infirmary and at Providence. The Daughters of Mercy created the Blessed Martin de Porres Hospital, still there; that's now the Allen Memorial Home on the corner of Washington Avenue and Virginia. Daughters of Mercy had this hospital which was for black patients and black doctors, a transitional hospital. Soon after integration it closed. The Daughters of Charity had built a facility, the Allen Memorial Home, in 1932, to care for unwed mothers and for the aged. It provided confinement for the mothers and adoption for the children. Later, as time progressed, pregnancy out of wedlock became more accepted and it was okay to place these mothers in the regular hospital wards for their deliveries. When that happened, the Allen Memorial Home closed. It was originally located on St. Anthony Street across from the City Hospital. Then it moved to behind the old Providence Hospital at the corner of Katherine and Center Streets. Later the Daughters of Charity reopened the Allen Memorial in the Blessed Martin de Porres Hospital building as a long-term-care facility.

I was in Washington, D.C., at the time the Mobile Infirmary came up to ask for funding from the Hill-Burton Act. Their goal was to gain funds from Hill-Burton for what is now the new Mobile Infirmary. Hill-Burton had told the Infirmary they could only get funds if they had an integrated facility. The Infirmary responded that the Blessed Martin de Porres Hospital in Mobile was segregated and they got funding. So the argument ran that they should give to the Infirmary, too. And they did.

During the fundraising, Mr. J. L. Bedsole had the capacity to determine what each physician could give from his practice. He told me my obligation was one thousand dollars. Charlotte said, how can we give them a thousand dollars when we don't even have a toaster? After we came back from the war, most of us didn't have any resources. Poor. But he ended up getting his one thousand dollars. I don't know what would have happened if you hadn't, but you didn't question it. You just said, "Yes, sir, of course," and gave him the money. Bedsole and Roberts wrote the ticket. But they had leadership, they had organizational talents.

When we got back after World War II, the Mobile Infirmary far exceeded the quality of care. The same things were claimed to be done at Providence Hospital, but they did not have the best staff. Mobile Infirmary had it. They had laboratory technicians and medical directors to satisfy the needs and requirements of the patients. I think the best thing that ever happened was when Providence Hospital changed their identity and moved its building. They had just spent I think thirty million dollars within the last twelve months, but they moved out of the old facility and abandoned it. They had a string of dark-complected population that plagued them. They really and truly were plagued. Katherine White-Spunner would not let them be admitted at the Infirmary at one point in time. The City Hospital and Providence both had areas where blacks were taken care of. But they got overburdened.

During a reconstruction of the face of Providence, a crack went through the building. The entire hospital had to be moved. They moved into the old Alan Memorial Hospital on Center Street and Katherine. They moved in and took over the Alan Memorial. There were three or four floors there and that was the substitute for Providence. In 24 hours they moved out and never broke stride. And why did that happen? Because it was run by dictators. Tight management got that sort of thing done.

The patient chose the hospital; that was the way. We had an open staff in Mobile. And the open staff gave you privileges of being on Blessed Martin de Porres, City Hospital, all the hospitals. The patient decided where they wanted to go. If they were Catholic, they went to Providence;

Jewish, they went to Mobile Infirmary. If we didn't see them at one place, you saw them at another. If you got kicked off the staff at one hospital, you had the others. And if you didn't keep up your records at Mobile Infirmary you might censored for it but you could go to another hospital. Then when you get your records done, you could come back and practice. It's always been that way.

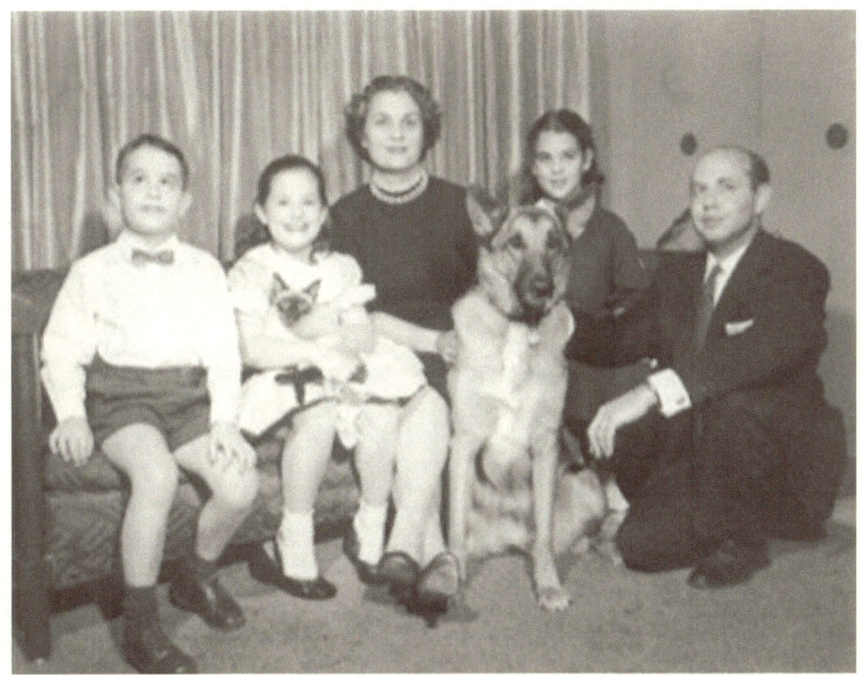

Dr. Samuel Eichold and Family in Mobile, Alabama, in the 1950s

We didn't have third-party reimbursement until the late sixties. Blue Cross came in. The mistake we made was we let Blue Cross Blue Shield write the contract and we had to agree to service the contract. And when they wrote the contract the doctors couldn't get together enough and say this stuff doesn't service our patients. We could have told them that we can't accept this. Instead we got stuck, because the doctors wouldn't get together.

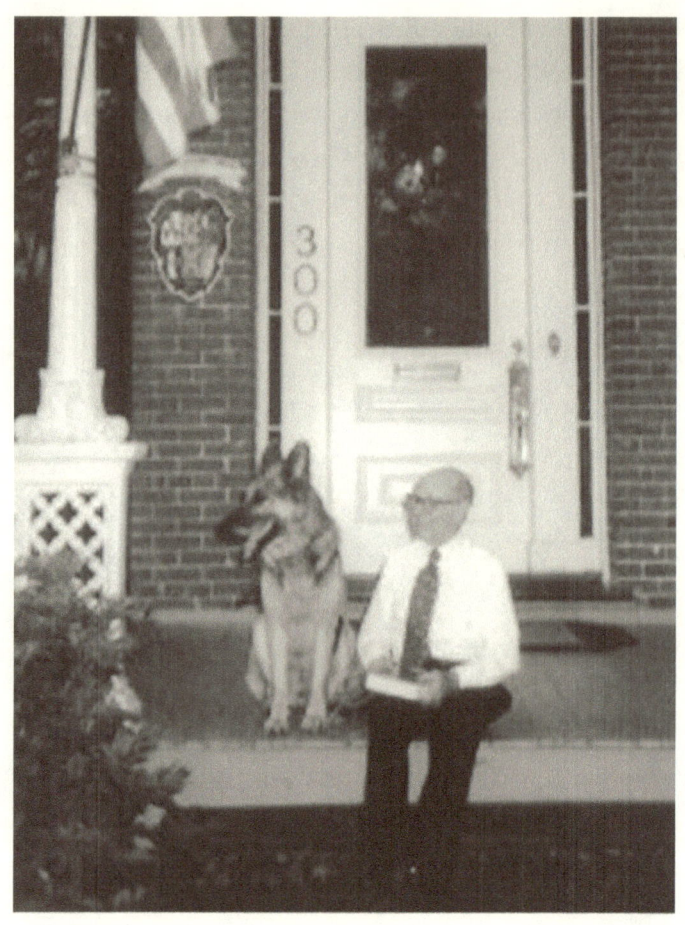

Dr. Sam Eichold II, professor emeritus of the University of South Alabama College of Medicine, at his home on Chatham Street (2000)

CHAPTER 9

M. Annelle Woodall Jerome, "Mama J" (1918–1999)

Wife of Dr. Shepard Jerome and Registered Nurse

Judson College 1940

Touro Infirmary Nursing School 1943

Dr. Shepard Jerome (1917–1990)

Harvard 1938

Tulane Medical School 1944

I am originally from Tallassee, Alabama. A little tiny country town, up close to Montgomery. I was born and raised on a farm and I did nothing but work on a farm the whole time I was in school until I graduated from high school and went off to college. I went to Judson College in Marion, Alabama. This was 1936. Way back there. I got a scholarship to go: a scholarship in music. Now, if you want me to tell you some real stories?

I grew up on a farm and my father was the kind of person that insisted that I learn how to work. So I had five hundred chickens, about five cows, and pigs and horses, you name it. But the chickens were my job. I had to feed them. I had to order the feed. I had to clean the roost. I had to collect the eggs. I had to sell the eggs. I had to take care of all the sick chickens. Well, as a teenager I didn't have too much social activities. I learned to love my chickens and I learned to sing with them. I was singing one day with the chickens and it upset them so that mother came down to the place and said what in the world are you doing? I said I'm teaching myself how to cackle and talk to the chickens. This is a long story . . .

I got to college and the freshmen had to put on an act. The first thing they said was that you've got to get on the stage and do something so that the whole school will understand and know who you are. Well, I had no talents other than learning to cackle like a chicken when I was working with chickens. I found a professor who had some chickens and so I borrowed one. I got this lady at the school to play on the piano *The Blue Danube*. So I dressed up like a hillbilly went out on the stage under the spotlight with my real chicken and put it down in front of me and I cackled to the tune of *Blue Danube*. Well, it scared that chicken so until he poo-pooed all over the stage. It scared him to death and everybody howled. And for the first time in my life I learned how to make a positive out of a negative. I looked at that chicken and laughed, picked it up, wiped up all the poo-poo and ran off the stage. Till this day, they have not forgotten my chicken act.

Well, all through the years, I've been able to use this chicken act. As a nurse—when I graduated from college I went into nursing down at Touro Infirmary in New Orleans—and as a nurse with all the children in pediatrics I was cackling and they all waited for the chickens to come on every day. When a person was coming out of an anesthetic, I would cackle and they wondered where in the world they had been when they finally woke up. I've had a lot of fun with my chicken. Now, I worked with a lot of internationals through all of these years. I have found that the chickens make the same sounds all over the world. So, with a lot of fun I've had the chicken episode over in Poland and over in Switzerland and over in Holland. And now, I am putting on a chicken act for all these senior citizens around here to teach them how to laugh again. I'm still enjoying my chickens. I have three different kinds of chicken cackles:

This is the one that is too old to lay an egg

The one that's too young to lay an egg

The one that is just right that learns to sing!

It boggles my brain. I'm known as the crazy lady with the chicken voice. That's the crazy side of me.

Now, being a nurse all these years, you have to learn how to laugh when there is sadness. And if you can bring a little joy and something to perk people up when they are in sorrow, then my chickens have come in real good and I learned all that.

I was a home economics major, and a minor in music and a minor in science. I had all my premed ready to go to med school. At that point in time they weren't taking too many girls into medicine. This was 1940. I went into nursing and I ended up teaching some of the same things I was supposed to be taking cause I had had all of my sciences. That was at Touro Infirmary in New Orleans and I graduated in '43. I met a medical student in 1941 and it was amazing. The same professors that taught at the medical school at Tulane were teaching at Touro. And so we were correlating our studies together and of course his was on a higher level than mine and we enjoyed each other as he went through medical school and I went through nursing. I graduated a year before he did. I stayed on and worked with Touro Infirmary until we got married the day he graduated from medical school in 1944. We were married then and this was during World War II: everybody was overworked and underpaid. You can't imagine what medicine was like at that particular time.

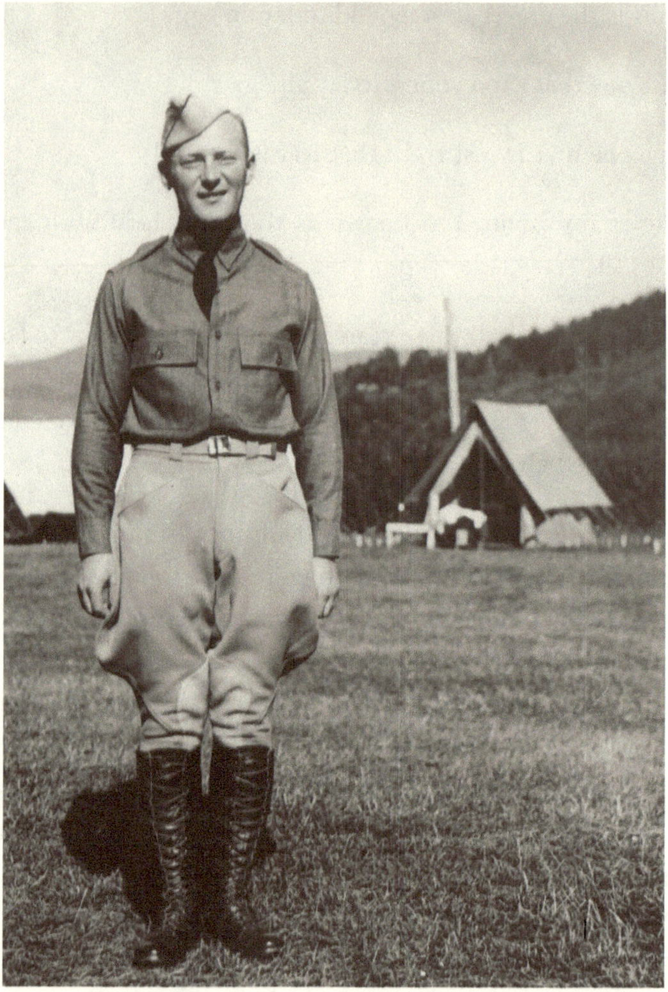

Shepard Jerome in the regular Army as a field artillery officer, where he served for two years, from 1938 to 1940, after graduating Harvard (undated photo)

Infection rates were still lower, but syphilis and gonorrhea was running rampant. All of the nurses, the RNs, were pulled out of the hospitals—and the doctors were pulled out—and they left all of us younger ones. There was nothing for me to have 40 patients a day. There was nothing for me to deliver a baby on the elevator. We had patients lined up in the halls. There was just no way that you could legally make a record of everything that was happening because there was not enough help. Its a thousand wonders we didn't have a lot more catastrophes than we did.

I was the very first nurse at Tulane Infirmary to give a shot of penicillin in 1942 in a pediatric ward to a child about ten years old. A miracle happened. It helped her and she overcame her illness immediately. It just looked like a miracle. We were all apprehensive. We were biting our nails, wondering if it was going to work.

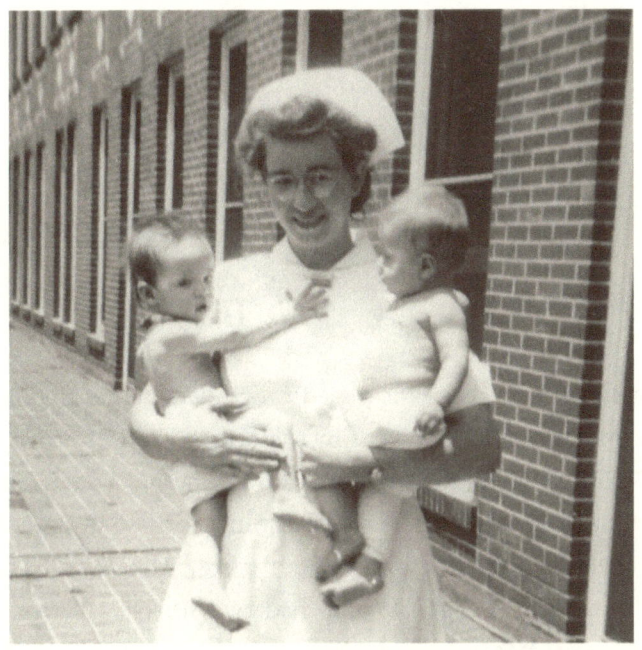

Annelle Woodall, RN, working in pediatrics at Touro Hospital,
New Orleans (1944)

The sterilizing procedures were archaic. We had to do all of our tubes, wash the tubes out and try to sterilize all the tubes that we used; everything. There was no such thing as disposable items, linens, nothing. We had to do all the laundry. I wore white stockings, white shoes, and white starched uniforms. And I said if I ever got out of all that stuff, I'd never put white stockings on again. I ate my words.

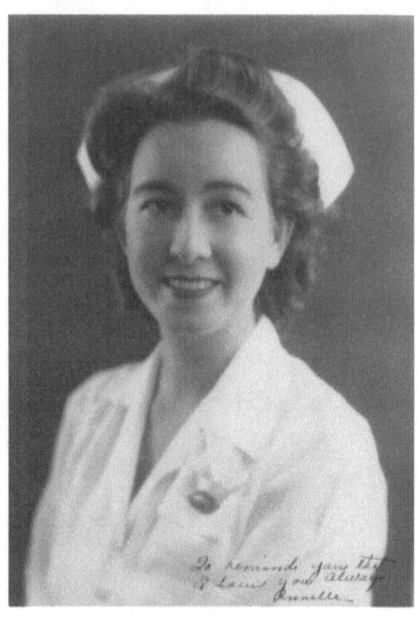

Annelle Jerome, RN (1944)

During the war, in order for a medical student to get his internship—and all the medical students were in the armed services, Army, Navy, or whatever—you were assigned to something whether you liked it or not. Dr. Shep was assigned to the Marine Hospital out in San Francisco for his internship. It took us four days to get out there on the train. There was no such thing as airline flying. We only had two suitcases between us. All I had was uniforms. When I got married, I had one suit, which was a black suit. The rest of my clothes were uniforms. Why, I hadn't owned anything other than uniforms for three years.

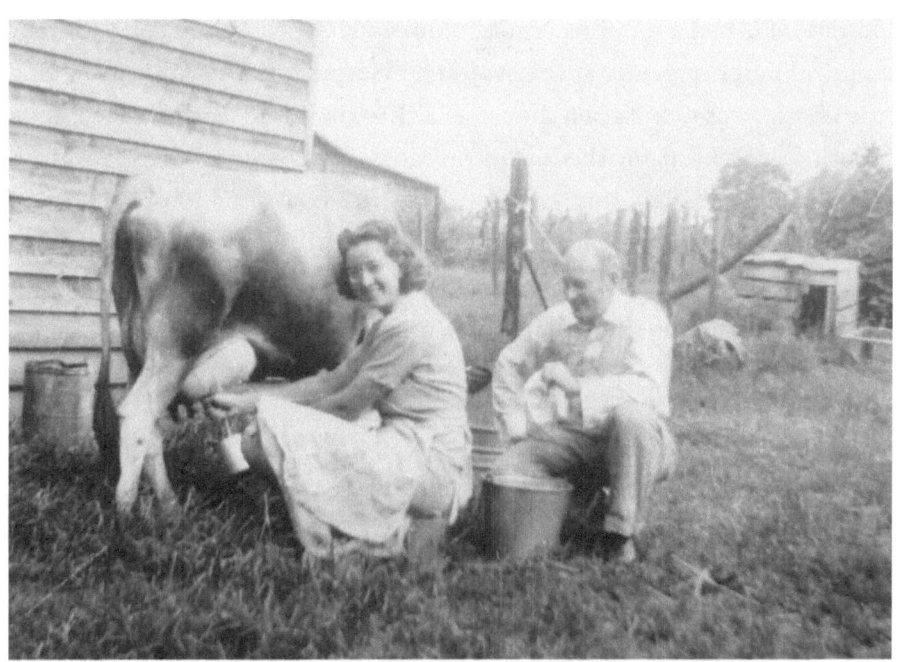

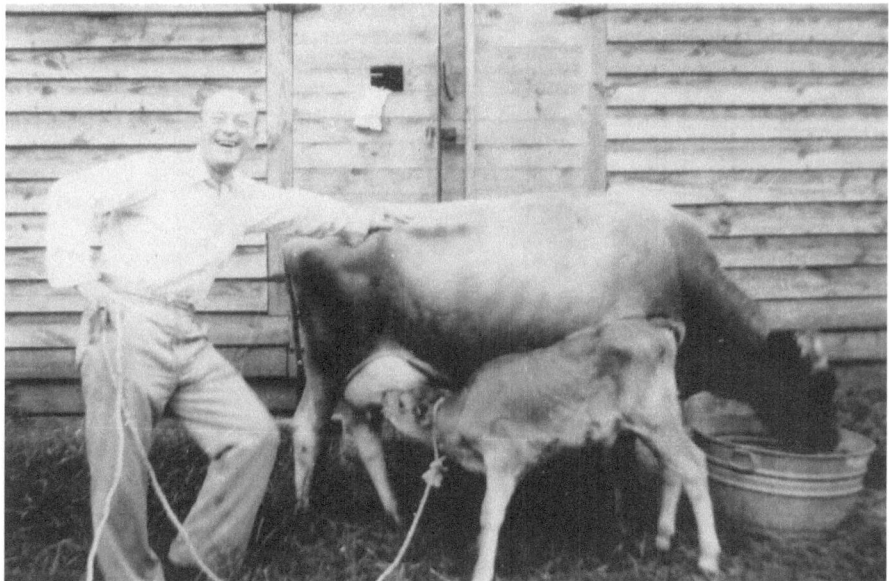

Shep and Annelle visiting Woodall family home in Tallassee, Alabama (1944)

We went out there and finally found us an apartment, which was really tough, because everything was full. Big base. He interned at the Marine

Hospital. He had a lot of real exotic things to happen to him. And for four months I taught nursing at the St. Joseph Hospital there substituting for a teacher who was sick. When she came back on I went to work for the Public Health Department for the rest of the time. Do you know what I was? A "chippie chaser." Have you ever heard of that? It was my job to run in all the prostitutes who had contracted with venereal disease. I walked into two or three murders. I'm in the process of writing all this down and including it in my book on the crazy life of a doctor's wife.

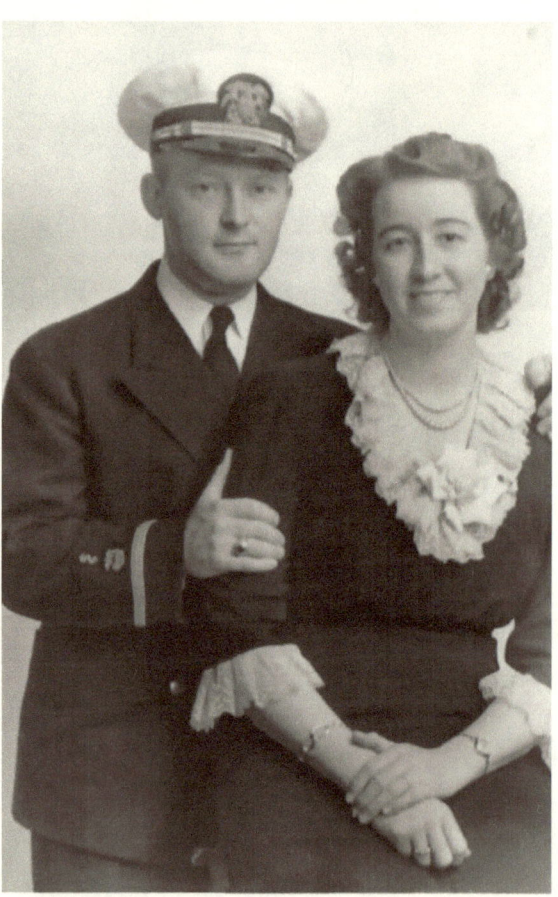

Annelle and Dr. Shepard Jerome in public health uniform, San Francisco (1944)

What was so funny was that down in New Orleans, at Touro, I had some time in the clinic down there and was running down the venereal disease contacts. In California I was also running the venereal disease contacts. I went to this black family, knocked on the door, and said that I was asking for Joe. Joe was there and he said "Lordy, Lordy, Lordy, Ms. Woodall! What you do all the way from New Orleans." I said, well, from New Orleans to California, you're bringing venereal disease, so come on in and get your shot.

Doc and I were involved in helping to catch a big criminal out there. He came home one night and told me that this guy had been into the Marine Hospital and he had a horrible case of venereal disease. He had a most peculiar tattoo on his arm. Well, I thought nothing about it. About three weeks later, I was running the clinic for venereal disease and in walks this man. In the meantime, Shep had come in the next week and said the FBI is looking for this guy all over because he is a murderer. Well, this guy came into the clinic and I recognized the markings on his arm.

I got to the back phone and called Shep. I said, "Tell me again what he looked like." And he described the gentleman sitting there and I told him that he was here. He said we'll call the FBI. I'll call the FBI; just try to hold him there. I got on the phone with the FBI and they told me to make sure that I got him in the back room and away from everybody and to clear everybody out cause he was dangerous. Long story, short ending. I got the doctor in the back and told him what was going on. He called the guy in and I cleared all the people out of the clinic. It wasn't too long before I heard the sirens coming and sure enough they went in and got him, and he was the one that they had been looking for. He had killed four people on his way from New York to California. It was an apprehensive time. This was in '44 and '45.

We were there finishing his internship. Then we were sent to Carlisle, Pennsylvania, for some of his specialty training. He had been in the regular Army before the war and he was in the field artillery for two years after he graduated from Harvard in 1938. He had been in ROTC at Harvard and he wanted to stay in. Well, nobody could get out then; this was still during the war. They gave him captain's rank, in the Army Medical Corps, and we went to Carlisle, Pennsylvania. While we were up there, I babysat, rather than nursing. I sat with a doctor's family taking care of all their kids, doing the cooking, cleaning, and everything else for five kids for the six months we were there.

Then he was transferred to Denver, Colorado, to do anesthesia at the hospital there. And I ran a tourist court. Instead of trying a get a license to do nursing in Colorado, I knew that we would be there for only seven or eight months. I was able to get into this tourist court. The lady came down with cancer of the breast and had to have surgery. So I ended up running her tourist court for her. They had rooms, a boardinghouse. I did that for the whole time we were there. Then we were sent to Temple, Texas, for him to do anesthesia. I babysat for a doctor's family there rather than trying to get a nursing license.

He went into urology. The general that was there was the urologist in charge of the hospital. They assigned Shep, finally, out of anesthesia to work with all the paralyzed, the paraplegics. We had over 120 paralyzed boys there; some of them were quadriplegic. He ended up bringing two or three of them home for the weekend in wheelchairs. We had a one-bedroom apartment, but they wanted to get away from everything. So I worked myself to death, going up there and working with them on the wards and then bringing them home for the weekend. First baby was born while we were there. Then from there he was sent to Japan. The war was over. Finally, the war was over!

He was there about five months before I got there. When I traveled over there it was June 1946. My baby was about three months old. That was hazardous. We had to go from Montgomery on a train to Seattle, Washington, and be there a week for orientation before we could be put on a ship. There were about ten thousand dependents on this ship and it took us about 18 days to get to Tokyo. The worst part of the whole trip: we nearly hit some of the floating mines. We had an emergency drill that lasted about five hours and all of us had to be on deck. I was on the side of the deck where they were using all the machine guns to explode all of these floating mines. There were about 12 of them that we nearly hit, going through this whole mine area. But thank God, we got through it without any going off. But it was real apprehensive.

Well, then we got to Japan. I had no idea what, where, when, or who and just found out we were going into the harbor. They told us that it would be about five hours before we got in. The boat had slowed down and all of a sudden I heard, "Mommy! Mommy!" coming down the hall. Shep had signed on with the ship to be one of the doctors to okay everybody going off! So he got on the ship before we got into the harbor. I had a grand reunion with him down on the bottom floor. It was great! After we got off the ship, we had a three-day travel on an open train to get down to the island of Kyushu in a little town called Beppu and that's where we were for a year and half.

It was on the ocean. I don't guess you could call it pretty. It was a typical Japanese village. We had an 18-room house; straw floors, paper doors, thatched roof. You name it, we had it. They assigned us five servants. None of them spoke English. Now all of this was part of reparation. The servants that we had became part of our family. One of the houseboys had been a kamikaze pilot and he came to work with the full understanding in his mind that he was going to kill us. Long story short—I taught him how to read, to write, and to speak English. When we left, he was publishing a newspaper. Five years after we left Japan I found out he had one of the largest newspapers on the island of Kyushu. He told us what his intent had been, but that he had changed his mind. He became a real close friend.

The other locals were standoffish at first. We had been told that we had to be very, very careful with all of the people cause they didn't know how we would be accepted. Nobody knew. We were the first dependents in there after the war. We didn't have a store. We didn't have a way to shop. There was a supply train that came down every four months with anything and everything that we needed on it in the way of canned foods, Kotex, any clothing. No such thing as milk. Nothing. I took over a six-months' supply of baby food with me when I went. When that was gone that was it. She learned to eat everything that we ate. She lived on rice just like we did. I could buy a one-hundred-pound sack of rice and all of our servants and we could live on it all month. The kitchen had a dirt floor in it and hibachis and we cooked on those until they finally got us a little tiny electric stove.

We weren't allowed to eat anything that was raised there or grown there because everybody used the "night fertilizer," they called it. Our house had three open pit toilets. Once a week they came with dippers and dipped everything out of the basins that were underneath. And they took it all out and used it on all their gardens and all their fields. We were not allowed to eat any of it.

We had dehydrated food at that time. What was a big problem for me was that Shep had this 350-bed hospital and he had no one in the kitchen. All the kitchen help had been sent back to the states. He had no one in the kitchen to cook. Thank goodness I had some experience in home economics. I was put in the field kitchen with all those field stoves to cook on. We had around two hundred in the hospital to cook for every day three times a day for the year and a half we were there. Finally, they got some sergeants to help me in the kitchen. But for a while I was carrying the whole thing by myself. I went to the hospital and we got us an Army cot and built a frame around it for Judy. Kind of like a fence around it. And I'd take her up to the hospital and put her in that when I was working. So it wasn't easy, believe me.

I saw him when he wasn't working with the patients. He was able to come home about two nights out of the week. The rest of the time he was there 24 hours a day. There was one other doctor. Just the two doctors. That's for five thousand troops; for a 350-bed hospital. We had an average of around two hundred patients most of the time. We had an epidemic of scarlet fever that came on and was real rough. All of the nurses, all of the corpsmen that were working there were transferred back to the states and they hadn't sent any new ones in. So, I had to just take GIs that didn't even know which end of the thermometer to use and teach them how to help care for the patients.

I got a real big citation from this General Eikelberger. I don't even remember where he was from or anything. He was pulling inspection on the hospital and he couldn't believe all the things I had been doing. When I got ready to leave he gave me a big citation because I worked myself to death in that area. Then we were transferred up to Osaka and he was in the 25th Division surgery. He had over twenty-five thousand troops under his care, with about four hospitals under his care. Kept him busy and it kept me busy. We were responsible for giving all of the dependents in that whole area their shots. Immunization shots. Instead of all of them going down to Osaka. We had a house way up on the mountainside, another 15-room house with five servants. And every weekend that they had to have shots, we would have what we call a "Stick-Up Party" at the house. They would all come to the house. He'd have two nurses and I would help with it. He'd have his sergeant and we would give them all of their immunization shots at the house. Sometimes as many as three hundred shots on a Sunday afternoon.

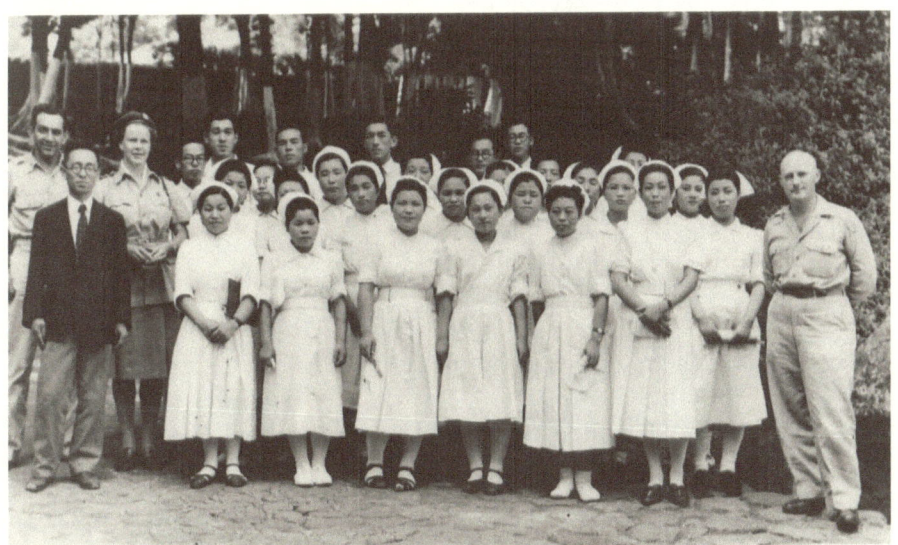

Dr. Shepard Jerome with nursing and hospital staff, Osaka General Hospital, Osaka, Japan (1947)

There in Kyushu, in Beppu, we were not too far from the second bomb area, Nagasaki. And the ones that survived soon found out that Shep was a doctor. We had this huge gate out front with steps coming up to it. When I would go out in the morning and there would be 15 and 20 people sitting on the steps moaning and crying, "isha, isha, isha, Doctor, Doctor." I got an interpreter to find out what they wanted. Some of them—the most gnarled-looking individuals you have ever seen: no eyes, some of them no ears, faces so deformed they couldn't even close their mouths. Hands like this. They had survived the atomic blast and had scar tissue everywhere. They were more concerned not about their physical being but about the fact that they were sterile and couldn't have a son. To them this was the most important thing in the world—to leave a son.

Shep organized a team of all of these Japanese doctors and we got all of these people going to a clinic that was run with the Japanese doctors. He had to oversee all of the clinics for the Japanese people. They didn't even have any of that after the war. So, he worked with this Dr. Nakamura out there in Beppu. Yeah, a long way from Tallasee, believe you me, from the chicken farm.

It was amazing. When I was growing up, our preacher at our Baptist church had been a missionary to Japan. He told me stories and I kept saying, Lord, some day I want to go to Japan. I didn't realize that I was going to be able to live there for three years, you know, and do all the work that I did. I taught nursing, taught cooking and sewing. And I went to the high school and gave them lessons in English. It was just a real challenge.

In the meantime, while I was there I took over about one hundred dollars worth of garden seed. Dug up my driveway and planted a garden. The general at the post almost put me in jail. I got my jeep, put a trailer on it, and went up to where all the horses were. I got some manure. And on the way back I was dropping manure along the road and he followed the droppings and found me. He said, "Don't you know what you're doing is illegal?" I said, well, the doctor in charge says it's all right. "If you get sick from any of this I'm going to be the first to send you home." Three months later, I had the most beautiful garden and there were eight American families there. We had nothing fresh. I was able to gather up my very first vegetables in a huge basket and I took them up to the general's house when I knew he was at home at lunchtime. Knocked on the door. I said, "General Yancy, I have something special for you." He looked at it and yelled, "Tomatoes! Where did you get them?" I said, "Sir, these came out of the garden with all the manure that I was hauling." "Next time you are hauling manure, if you'll just let me know, I'll let some of the GIs haul the manure for you." I furnished all of our families with fresh vegetables out of my garden.

A real ironic thing happened. We had to leave. And I had to leave my garden. We were transferred up to Osaka. All these years I wondered what ever happened to my garden because I had watermelons, cantaloupes. It was growing so beautifully. And I want you to know—this was about 15 years ago—a Chinese doctor here in Mobile asked us for dinner and there was another couple. This other guy had been a colonel in the Army and he and Shep started talking and we found out that both of us had lived in Beppu. I asked him where did you move to, what unit? We found out that they were the ones that moved into our house and acquired our garden. I couldn't believe it. And they told me that all the time they were there they had fresh vegetables out of the most wonderful garden they had ever seen. Can you believe that? My garden! I just get goose bumps. That is neat, unbelievable.

Now talking about the clinical: I had the nurses from Osaka and from Tokyo to come down because Beppu was sitting on top of a volcano. We had these hot sulfur springs coming out of the ground and everybody wanted to come down. We had one of those in our house and everybody wanted to come down to our house. When I'd meet them at the train station and say, "Come on, do you want to go to my house and take a bath?"

I took them on tours of the hospital and, of course, we got to know all the Japanese doctors. Surgery then was unbelievable in the hospital there at Beppu. This was typical of the operating room: They had five tables. They had two people at each table. I took a tour of nurses through and we didn't have to put on a mask or gown or anything. The floor was all wet. Here was a table with instruments on it and this was a case with infection here. And this one at another table was doing a hysterectomy. They were swapping instruments back and forth. If we had ever done that in America we would have been hung by our ears, you know. They didn't give anesthesia. This lady, I stood at her head and she was having this hysterectomy. I asked her if it was hurting and she said, "No, no," and the sweat was just pouring off of her. She was cringing with pain. They are so stoic. I wanted to help her so badly. There was nothing you could do. The nurses that were with me were cringing too. And here was this guy who had a real bad leg that had been split open and they were working on that and taking sharing instruments off the same tables. I couldn't believe it.

I took one of the maids that we had to have a mastoidectomy. And I went with her to the hospital and stayed with her. Now this is in '46. Your patients had to have the family to go with you, take your bed, take your hibachi to do your cooking, take anything and everything that you would need the whole time that you are there. They are put on the floor. I stayed with her in surgery. They gave her nothing and did a mastoidectomy and finally she fainted away. I was hoping and praying that she'd hurry and faint from the pain so that she would be out of it. I brought her home the next day and she was an invalid in our home for about a week before she could finally get up and go. But the trauma of all that without anesthesia is I think as bad as the pain. It's unbelievable.

They had no medicine. None. What Shep would do, when he finally got penicillin in the hospital over there, he would save the empty bottles and use some sterile water and rinse the bottles out. We had a family way up in the country and they came just begging Shep, "My husband is dying, please he needs some antibiotics and we know that you've got it." Well, he used some of the washings out of the penicillin bottles and went up there and gave the guy these shots. It cured him. I've got two pictures hanging in my den in yonder that those people gave us because Shep cured the man.

We came back the fall, October of '48. We were stationed in Augusta, Georgia, at the hospital there. We were there about a year and half and then they closed that hospital. Then they sent him to San Antonio, Texas, to work down there. I had to close up the house and do all the moving, do everything. This general that he got to know insisted that he stay in the Army and get a urological certification. So he was appointed to the urology department and he did his five years in urology there. San Antonio. Then, we were sent to Fort Benning, Georgia, after that.

Dr. Jerome was from Boston. A Yankee stumped his toe on a Southerner and stayed down South! Well, anyway, we were there until 1955. He was scheduled to be sent to Europe. He had moved around—we had moved around so much. We had two children at the time and they were at the stage of getting ready to go to school. He said I'm ready to get out. He had had 17 years of regular Army then. So he decided, we prayed about it, and he decided to come to Mobile. This is where we ended up in 1955.

Picked it out of the hat, really. He was offered partnerships in Denver, Colorado, San Francisco, and Montgomery, Alabama, and San Antonio. They all wanted him to come join them. He had Army friends that had gotten out in all of these areas. They knew him and they all wanted him. We came down to Mobile and looked things over and we both prayed about it and we just felt like this is where the Lord wanted us. So this is where we ended up.

And it was really rough. When we got here, I established the office and then I went to work for Mobile Infirmary. I taught nursing at the Mobile Infirmary. And I was the PR person for the school of nursing there. Then I ran the office and did all the surgery with him in the office. You name it, we did it. We did it together. He finally got on top of it all. He stayed in urology until 1982, and he was by then burned out on surgery, he had done so much. And so he wanted to give up his urology practice. He became the medical director of Providence Hospital. Their very first medical director at the old Providence: he was on the ground floor of helping to plan the new building. And to plan all of the facility and all of the framework of the organizational part of the nursing and the medical offices.

We had a strong spiritual bond. Dr. Jerome was an Orthodox Jew. For the three years we dated, he didn't tell me anything about it. He went to church with me as a Baptist. He told me he was Methodist. Three hours before we were married he broke down. The night before he got a call from his father and he promised his daddy that he wouldn't marry me until he told me. Well, three hours before we were married he finally broke down and told me.

He didn't want to tell me because if you remember in the 1940s, this was when the Jews were so unpopular. He had been ostracized the whole time he was growing up because he was Jewish. Anti-Semitism was strong, very much so, especially up in lower Massachusetts, in Boston, where he was raised. He had a lot of friends that were Catholic and he would try to go to church with them and because he was Jewish, they wouldn't let him in.

Then when he finished Harvard and two years in the regular Army, all his buddies knew his background. And all the officer's clubs—no blacks and no Jews allowed. So he was ostracized many times. When he came down South he knew how Southerners were. When he came to Tulane to medical school, he was determined not to let anybody know his heritage. Well, finally he told me. He said, "There are two things that I'm going to say: I'm Orthodox Jew so don't cram your religion down my throat, and my profession will always be first." He said, "Is this going to make any difference?"

And I said, "Well, I can tell you frankly, I have prayed over this very, very long and I didn't pick you out—God picked you out for me, because if I'd been picking you out it would have been a guy as tall as me, with hair, and no false teeth!" He was bald when I met him. He said he lost his hair his first year at Harvard, he studied so hard. He had two front teeth that were false. It made no difference with us.

The six years after we were married, everywhere we'd go I'd go to church. Sometimes it would be an Episcopal church, a Catholic, whatever church was there. He would always go with me. But he would never let me discuss it. But he went with me when we were stationed in San Antonio, Texas. He went with me to a revival meeting one night. The sermon was, "Christianity Is for the Jew as well as the Gentile," and he realized that Jesus is the Messiah and without saying a word to me he walked down and accepted Jesus as his Savior.

He was the most dynamic Christian you could ever find. He knew the Old Testament and studied the New Testament. He could correlate everything with the Old Testament and it was unbelievable. He was just a dynamic Christian. You know, all these years clearly his medicine came first, that's true. But now the first year after he died I kept saying, you know I'm still mad—not at him—but at medicine, because it just usurped him so much that he was so engulfed in medicine. And then I started getting letters from all over the world: "I wouldn't be the doctor today that I am if it hadn't been for Dr. Jerome." People in just every walk of life write me a letter or call me long-distance. "I want you to know that Shep meant more to me than you could ever know because he begged me to understand Christianity." I understand how God used him through his medicine to be His witness. I can not be angry at a profession like that. Thank goodness, being a nurse, I understood where he was coming from. His dedication to his patients was unparalleled to anybody that I have ever known. He had always wanted to be in medicine. He finished Harvard in premed and he just focused on it. He felt like this is what he was supposed to do in life. A gut feeling that this is what he had to do.

CHAPTER 10

Edwin Chandler "Pete" Bramlett, Sr. (1919–2000)

Hospital administrator

University of Mississippi 1940

Business Manager of Mobile Infirmary Medical Center, 1949

Administrator of MIMC 1959, retired in 1984 (35 years)

Interviewed in June 1994 at 75 years old

The sixties were wonderful. Well, we had in the medicine and health care operation in Mobile—we had a ideal setup. The County Medical Society was split two ways. One was with the Providence Hospital which was Catholic. The other was Mobile Infirmary which was for Protestants and Jewish. Then there was the St. Martin de Porres Hospital which was for blacks. Then a City Hospital took care of all the indigent. Poor, black and white. We had no real indigent problem as far as running the Mobile Infirmary was concerned. We had no doctor problem because the doctors were members of all three medical staffs, but they had their primary notice of where they belonged up front. You knew who exactly was a Providence doctor, who was a Mobile Infirmary doctor.

Allegiances were identified right off the bat. You knew exactly who to support, exactly who to listen to, exactly who to follow through with the medical staff. Then on top of that, we had just finished, in '52, a five-year drive where the churches and the doctors and the community business played a part in raising two million dollars for the new Infirmary.

Our Board of Trustees were made up of two Baptists, two Episcopalians, two Methodists, two Presbyterians, one Christian, one Lutheran for a total of 14 board members or so of that nature. They appoint them for a three-year term so we had to go to the congregation and suggest to them the names that we would like to have on the Board. We may or may not get them. So that maintained a high end of the churches with the hospitals because they were religiously involved. The Baptists were involved and became a real source of admission of patients. There were very few Catholic patients. They were going to the Catholic hospitals.

We moved out here to Springhill Avenue in 1952. We were still seg-regated. I had come on in '49. Well actually, what happened, Kathryn White-Spunner asked the Board of Trustees if they knew of anybody that could come. Sonny McRae was president of Merchant's National Bank and suggested my name. So I came by way of the bank and the bank told me they'd give me my job back if I didn't like it out there. But I came into it because for three generations before me there had been doctors in our family and I couldn't go into medical school. I was in med school for three years, University of Pennsylvania, but I had to drop out because my father got paralyzed from an automobile accident. So I took business administration, University of Mississippi, which was our home originally. My father, when he practiced medicine, graduated first from the University of Pennsylvania. So he opened his practice up in Philadelphia.

Got to Mississippi, graduated in 1940 and married a Mobile girl in 1941. Worked for IBM when I graduated. I was one of three selected out of the southeastern area with IBM, worked with them until the war came. Then I went in—I was a commissioned officer in the Navy. Yeah, I'll tell you I was a hot shot!

I was at a football game when Pearl Harbor was bombed, in Charlotte, North Carolina, with IBM. I was sitting at the first professional football game I ever saw and they announced that Pearl Harbor had been bombed. At halftime the game stopped. I wasn't enlisted then. I had made application for a commission in the Army at that particular point in time, but that never came through. Then I made application for the Navy and I went over to New Orleans to take the examination. There was a whole room full. I took the examination. They asked for two people to stay and I was one of the two that stayed. They put me through a battery of tests. Told me to get over there at 8:00 in the morning. I stayed inside; I had all sorts of written examinations and oral examinations until 6:00 that night. I came out enlisted in the United States Navy. My wife was sitting out there waiting the whole time, wondering what happened to me. I got my commission two months later.

They needed someone to work the IBM machine, so that was my great thing. I thought I was coming to run a PT boat and ended up working an IBM machine. Then I got assigned to Trinidad, to one of the offices down there. The day after VE-Day my wife and son joined me down there. It was pretty, pretty nice. So I couldn't fuss with PT assignment. After the war (around '46) I thought I was depressed about it because here I was a lieutenant commander and I go back to the Merchant's National Bank and do a little work that a high school graduate could do. So when the opportunity came to come to the hospital, I jumped at it.

I came to the old hospital (Mobile Infirmary) in '49 and there was no business organization at all. I mean they were hand posting everything and some things were left off. And depending on who you were, they would scratch them off and what have you: no charges and things of this nature. So I put in a NCR, national cash register, system, which was the window posting we used on most hospitals, hotels then. They would post the room charge, then your other charges for your drugs and surgical services, oxygen and so forth. It was established in other areas, we were just slow getting started to it. That stayed with us for a number of years, window posting did, until we finally got a little bit on the computer. It was a cash type of business. You paid for what you got. If you couldn't pay for it, we would try to collect it. If we couldn't collect it, we would write it off. But most of the patients could pay. And the doctors admitted patients who paid the hospitals. The ones who couldn't pay, they went to the City Hospital. Insurance wasn't a thing at all. You paid your doctor and he charged what he thought you could pay. Or you'd send him a chicken or two. Some folks would do that.

175 beds. One charge. The bill came in as a whole operating room charge. The anesthesia was separate and the physician charges were separate. Then they came in later on with an assistant physician charge, which we collected for them. The supplies were reusable, you had to resterilize them, resterilize the drapes, gloves, and everything else. It was a pretty good procedure. We had no disposable sponges. We used things of that nature. We used a lot of these lap sponges, used over and over again, sterilized, washed, and sterilized.

Mrs. White-Spunner was a marvelous person. Yeah, she knew that she had no expertise in the business or the purchasing and things of that nature so she immediately delegated that all to me and gave me one hundred percent freedom to do with [it] what I wanted to do with it. Yeah, and personnel as well. I had it all and then of course, some of the accounting. I got Milton Booth on board. He came from Turner Supply out there. He was an outstanding accountant. He graduated from Springhill College in accounting. He did a real good job, stayed with me for all the years I was here. He retired about six years ago. We really had a loyal staff. That's what I'm saying. In the sixties there was a situation: we didn't have any personnel turnover. I mean, it was just constant; the same old folks was all involved in it. And we put in certain procedures.

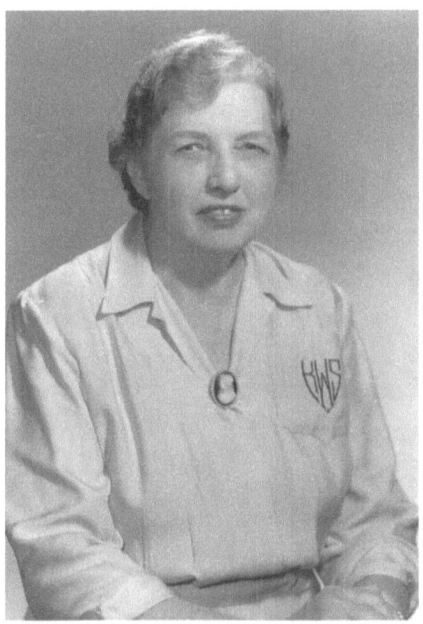

Ms. Katherine White-Spunner (1959) From Harry Webster: "She had enough presence so that she was able to control a cantankerous bunch of doctors."

I'm talking about the whole works of hospital management. When the proprietary hospitals came in, that started the competition and they started bidding for personnel. See Providence had its own school of nursing; we had our own school of nursing. So we replaced our personnel with our graduates. So we had no personnel shortage because we were bringing our own graduates in and we were working student nurses. Student nurses worked on the floors in a nursing capacity. They got on-hands training. They didn't just go to the classroom. They went on the floor which saved us some personnel money right off the bat.

Well, the only way the proprietary hospitals could get help was to buy it. The bidding wars began with proprietary hospitals. The proprietary hospitals made the first move. It was that group out of Nashville: Hospital Corporation of America. They started and of course we didn't do nothing but match it and then it started. It spread through all the whole area. The loyalties began to depend upon who gave 25 dollars a month more rather than the fact that you worked there all your life.

We put in a pension plan; we paid the insurance, life insurance, other things to hold people. We put in a very good pension plan. It's still a very effective one today. In 1952 or '53, I started the pension plan and Mr. Bedsole said, "No, you don't want a pension plan." Mr. McRae said yes. Mr. McRae and I won. That was the first real perk we had and group life insurance. Health insurance didn't come along until a later period, maybe seven, eight years later. Those were the main perks we had: the group life insurance, pension plan, and the health insurance.

We had, I guess in the early fifties, put in a group life insurance, five thousand dollars per person. We had one black man die in the laundry. His wife worked in laundry as well. So we gave her the five-thousand-dollar check and we asked her what she was going to say about it, she said, "Well, when I get married again, I'm marrying a Mobile Infirmary nigger!" Oh yeah, that was one of the little stories that come along. The blacks were extremely loyal. In fact, I can walk through the halls here now and more blacks will speak to me than whites will. I tried my best and succeeded to be fair to all of them. They knew they could count on me. They knew they could walk in my office as well as you could. They did, too. I went down to the jailhouse many times on Saturday to get a couple of them out of jail. I went to their funerals. They called me a benevolent dictator. You had to be a dictatorship to get the work done. That's the most efficient way, a dicta-torship. A benevolent one helps a little. Well, you've got to know who is boss and who to listen to. You can't have a divided segment: who is gonna be the president and who is gonna be the head of something. You've got to have one person who is responsible and they know that if they go to see you, they know you'll give them an answer. That's the answer; that's what it's gonna be.

The way we handled suggestions . . . if someone had any idea or wanted anything, they would bring it up to us, go up the ladder through the organ-ization and would come right to the top where the final decision was made unless the authority had been delegated to a department head or some-one else. Any policy things would come right up to me and I would take them to the board. Most nonpolicy decisions that were not handled by department heads, I would handle them. In fact I can't comprehend now the number of vice presidents they have here. I mean, it's a bloc of them. I think two of us, three of us ran the hospital for so many years and now they've got so many extra people. We started the new Infirmary at 285 beds and additionally over the years we got 750 beds. There aren't 750 beds now. We had 750 beds with 100 percent occupancy. With a staff of about two thousand. By then management was about five with department heads. It has changed because of outside interference.

It was a personal touch, a freedom, a personal feeling of relationship. We built on that. That was part of our strength. Our personnel was part of our real strength. We all had a good time, we really did. Sharing each other's problems, each other's joys. I can't think of anything more to say about it other than the fact that you've got a very different type of situation now because of outside interference and outside is a big world. The one area which we had evolved in was union activities and so forth: we were able to refuse union activities by maintaining a personal contact with our employees; the unions never got off the ground down here.

Well, first of all, they came in with Blue Cross. Blue Cross came in with certain requirements as to how you can be eligible for Blue Cross. That made us have to put on a certain staff person to handle the Blue Cross; Blue Cross made sure they got paid. Following that Medicare came. Medicare brought all the federal regulations in and all the state, city, and county regulations came flying in, so we had to employ extra people to comply with all these regulations. And that started us putting them between the patient and the Mobile Infirmary. We had this great big barrier of insurance. Outside insurances: we couldn't deal directly with these patients anymore. We had to go through these other parties. That's what changed the philosophy and brought so many extra people on board.

Then personnel came in and we couldn't hire and fire as easy as we could in the past situations. I had several personnel suits filed against me for firing people. I had one: We were the first hospital to start an intensive care area and coronary care unit as well. We had two units up there and there was a black LPN [licensed practical nurse] in this unit over here and they needed help over here and they asked her to come over and help and she wouldn't do it. She said that's not my station. So I fired her the next morning. But I got a suit filed against me for it. We won the suit. I think we paid off one, once.

I did a lot of the purchasing. All the salesmen came to see me; all the detail men would come to my office first. To see me first. I worked six days a week. I make my rounds at nighttime, three to 11 and 11 to seven every two months. I would do that so they could see me and know me and I could visit with them at the nursing station. Otherwise, they felt isolated because here at 5:00 p.m. everybody walks off the job. I found out that I learned more from the salesman about new products and things to do; learned more about the operation of the hospital from the people; they'd tell me these things. They were right there.

By 1946, the community was starting to grow a little bit and the bed shortage was quite obvious. But you couldn't do anything during the war with it. They had beds in the corridors. Catherine White-Spunner, who was the administrator then, or director of nurses she was called then, went with some of her board members—Mr. Bedsole, Mr. A. Roberts, and Mr. Penny McRae—and said they wanted to build a new hospital. So Bedsole then said he'd dedicate a year of his life to raising the money for it. He dedicated a whole year of his business to do it. He didn't have that much. He just had one secretary.

He was smart with money, in timber and other areas. He was pretty individually wealthy, so we had some help. He had owned an old department store in Thomasville, Grovehill, Jackson, and Fairhope. Yeah, he was quite a man. He was a dictator, without the word benevolent in front of it. He was tough. He wouldn't pay anybody any money. That's how he got a lot of it, from personnel. I started to work here for 150 dollars a month.

I had to keep up with the Hill-Burton grant which we got and all the accounting had to be done for that. And the purchasing: making sure all the purchases were proper, what discounts were given—there was no funny business going on. I had to keep all the records. I kept most of all those on a hand record book. I maintained all of that and did the purchasing for the new addition. We bought Simmons furniture throughout: Simmons mattress, Simmons furniture.

We realized the big thing was the payment of bills. When Blue Cross came in you had an insurance company paying bills so a lot of your collection work went down the drain because you didn't have to worry with it because Blue Cross paid for it. For collections, it was on a cash basis only; you had to try to collect from people who wouldn't pay their bills. We would turn them over to bill collecting agencies. They would do all sorts of threats and so forth of that nature just to collect the bill, courtroom suits and all the rest of that. We got 50 percent of what they collected. We tried to collect it ourselves for about six months, before we'd turn it over to them.

For the fund-raising Bedsole got all the churches and all the preachers in by having the churches organized, you see. Each church had their own goals. They raised money from its congregation out of its annual budgets and they had a five-year pledge from all the Baptists in town, Episcopal and all the rest of them. Yeah, all the churches were involved in making contributions. Oh, he was good. He met with the Ministerial Association and talked to them about it and it was quite obvious. I mean Mobile was in bad shape.

Building the new hospital was a challenge, very satisfactory. Personally you could see something going on, developing, growing with it. It wasn't a job for me. I just loved it. I came here in the morning, fresh and vigorous. I left in the evening tired. It was really a joy; it wasn't a job at all. I mean I had it in the same basis I had my family in. It was good. It had to be because of the amount of money they were paying me at that particular point in time. I could have gotten, I got some offers from other jobs to go somewhere else but I didn't want to leave Mobile because my wife's family was here. I moved mother and father down from Opp, Mississippi. They were here too, so our roots were getting pretty deep here in Mobile.

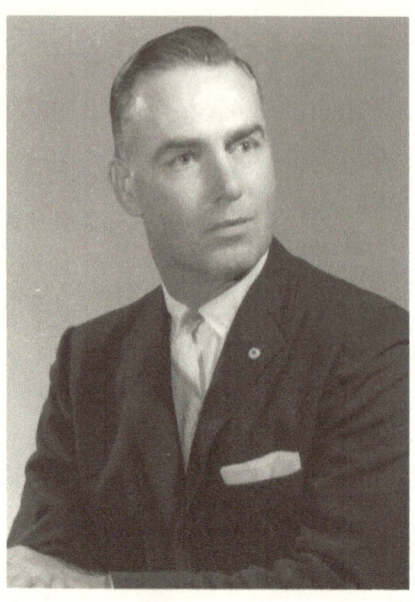

E. Chandler Bramlett (1959)

We had the big drive which financially got us all started. Once we got built, we didn't need any financing for a while for construction or anything. Then we built the nursing home over there by the nursing school building. I've forgotten the year that was built now, at least '50, I think. Now Dr. Abel's office and all that was nursing school dormitory and we built that on a low-interest loan we got from the federal government: two-and-a-half-percent interest loan. We built that and had a school of nursing and maintained a real fine school of nursing in the fifties. It was always filled with the number of students that we wanted, we could select.

Back in the years around the war there was a clique that ran the Medical Society and they wouldn't give anybody a license to practice unless they approved of them themselves. So you couldn't get in the Medical Society of the county unless this elite group approved you. So there was a number of doctors who tried to get in and couldn't get in. Ernie DeBakey was one of them; he was rejected initially. When they finally got that cleaned out, all the good doctors came in. I guess 1949, '50, '51, '52, for a number of years; we got some real good doctors in the Mobile area.

All the hospitals knew each other's territory and we abided by it. If we had any particular things we wanted to talk about, we would talk about it. But that doesn't necessarily mean we would agree on it. It was very difficult to deal with the sisters because their rules and regulations were coming from St. Louis and they felt that we weren't carrying our fair share of the black patients. Which we were not, we were an all-white hospital. But there was the City Hospital and there wasn't a black hospital around. They had a lot of blacks at Providence. Oh yeah, somewhere in the seventies a lot of the Catholics started coming to the Infirmary because the blacks were so big at the Providence hospital. Yes, there were a lot of blacks down there during the fifties. No, they were not a segregated hospital. We, the Infirmary, were one of three or four in the whole United States that was segregated, a large size.

Mobile City Hospital or Mobile County Hospital or Mobile General, one of the three names, at that particular point in time; the nuns backed out of managing the City Hospital in the fifties. They were still down there then. They couldn't get any financial support from the city to help run it. The city didn't have any revenue for them. And so they leaned more heavily upon their own Catholic order to supply them the extra money to maintain a hospital. It finally got to a point that it was a real burden to the Church and the Church said they couldn't support that anymore. So then it changed from City Hospital to County Hospital. Then the County Hospital had it for a while and then it changed to University of South Alabama later on. We had local area hospitals, administrator groups, City Hospital, Providence, and St. Martin as well as ourselves. They opened Doctors Hospital next. That was done by Dr. Tucker and a few others that were involved with that one. Then Springhill Hospital opened. We became more competitive. I tried to build our own staff stronger.

After Blue Cross got started, commercial insurance came in too. A lot of the industries in this area, the large industry, the paper mills and the State Docks and Alabama Dry Docks, they all had insurance for their fringe benefits. Before insurance you had to be really sick to want health care. Now you have a lot of people just coming to see the doctor because it's a nice social visit. You really had to be sick before you came into the hospitals. It wasn't like a fire insurance policy. You used your health insurance. You don't want to use your fire insurance policy because you don't want your house to burn down. But you want to use your health insurance because you got it, so you use it.

They, the physicians, went along with it. They had to because their income was tied to it as well. They may be hollering about Medicare and so forth and not paying their full bills, but they're doing pretty good. We had no real competition between any of the hospitals. And the doctor was the kingpin. He admitted the patients so you had to play up to him all the time. Now it's the same except the loyalty of the doctors is not there. We had that once. Because I could depend on them. I knew which doctors I could talk with to do things for me. I knew when doctors came to say something to me; the ones I would really listen to were the certain ones in a certain category.

Well, there was three or four of them that were real good. Grady Seagrest was good; Bart Adams was good; Joe Little was good; Socrates Rumpanos was good, he was a partner of Joe Little. June McCafferty and James Donald were some of the ones in different areas of surgery. The laboratory was small, it was run by Dr. Wise and Dr. Wert and it was a real small thing. Dr. Wert came from the University of Pennsylvania down here and he developed one of the first in-house staff training programs. He had a pathology conference every Monday morning and doctors would come in there frequently. He was one of the first ones as far as medical on-site training. Ghost surgery went out the window: every tonsil that was taken out, the pediatrician came in and assisted taking out the tonsil. So he got 10 dollars for assisting and the anesthesia service was paid out, just for assisting the doctor.

If you graph these developments you could show it was just continuing to improve all the way through. Until recently, I really think now though that the attitude of the public, attitude of doctors, attitude of personnel is more of a "what can you do for me" rather than "what I can do for you." I don't think that there is the same loyalty amongst the employees as there was. I think that they have gotten into this maze of outside influence from labor laws, from Medicare regulations, from how you file a claim, from how you do this and all the stuff that is coming out of Washington. Bureaucratic red tape has put the employees in a competitive position for their wages, determined other than by management. Management doesn't have the personnel control and so personnel doesn't have the relationship with management. It's not a one-on-one basis anymore. Too many outside influences that get involved.

The quality of patient care probably hasn't gone down any, but the quality of how people think about it has. And there are more people that are more willing to sue now. There are more people willing to find fault with their doctor now. There are more people willing because they do not have a personal relationship with them. I think the personal relationship is one of the areas that keep people, from feeling close to you. A lot of that disappeared when they find you have third-party payment. Then they developed certain hours a week that they were gonna work and they worked those hours and they don't work the other hours.

I don't think I would have changed anything. I really don't. I think when we had problems we worked at them long and hard and the final outcome was what we expected, what we wanted. We knew for example that we were going to have to admit black patients. But it was a question of being able to time admission with the acceptance of everybody else. The doctors and the community, too. Because you see the patients: at that particular time, the social environment was that if you got in bed within a twin bedroom with a black patient, you got moved out. The rooms were segregated. Then that became an issue. They said you could not ask the color of the patient at the time of admission. I know that. They were assigned wherever they could go at that particular time and if they got in with a white person they didn't like, the white person would move out or the black one would move out. It was a big problem with 20 two-bedroom, semiprivate rooms. They had the same thing happening in Detroit but the point was they were not under the gun like the South was. In fact, there is more segregation now in Detroit than there is here in Mobile, Alabama.

The whole area was going through change, it wasn't just Mobile Infirmary. The whole social chain, everything was being changed. Well, I guess accepting change on anybody's part is difficult at times. It was difficult for the community, it was difficult for the individuals and they had segregated offices for example, the doctors did. Waiting rooms. In fact that was one of the things that HEW [Health, Education, and Welfare] told us . . . that we couldn't admit doctors to our staff who used segregated waiting rooms. We told them we were not going to do that. So we had to call for a hearing in Washington, D.C., trying to make us eliminate doctors from our staff who had segregated waiting rooms. We won, we found out, we proved the fact that we didn't have control over the doctor's offices—we had control over the doctor when he came to the Infirmary, but we didn't have any outside that. So we won that case.

I don't think we had any black nurses. We had them in the service areas. It changed when they finally became academically qualified for it. It took a period of time because they weren't. We had another suit on the school of nursing about not having any black students, so we were called in for that. We told them that we didn't have any qualified ones for them and they said oh yes you do and so we produced all the examinations we had. The National League of Nursing, from New York State, graded all the examinations. The examinations showed that there were none of them qualified. Then they said you ought to admit them because they don't have a good secondary school system down here. So we said we're not going to reduce our standards of care. So we won that one, too. Then I had some student nurses being admitted to Providence Hospital who were black and we had some of them that qualified, so we admitted them. Once they graduated, they came on the staff as nurses and so forth. But that was over a period of years.

Ultimately it wasn't that much of a shift because day to day you are living it and so you would change a little bit each day and not really realize you were changing. I became less autocratic because a lot of the shots were being called outside of our own organization. Our board of trustees didn't have the complete power that it had before setting policy because policies were being set from outside organizations that were reflecting directly on our operation here. When you have regulations coming in from Washington you either comply with those regulations or you aren't approved.

Ours was primarily a situation where we were not accepting Medicare patients because they wouldn't pay for them. The government wouldn't pay for them because we were an all-white hospital. Said we were segregating against the blacks. We finally passed a resolution that we would admit black patients. Then the doctors did not admit black patients to us so we were still segregating. A lot of them still wouldn't admit blacks here or they would admit them to the Providence Hospital and not here. That's why Providence moved out when they moved to Springhill. Because they were getting so many black patients to them from the area where they were that they were having a lot of their good white patients come over to us because they didn't want to be down there with all those blacks. They won't admit that. But that quite obviously was the hidden agenda behind it all.

I'd get calls from the NAACP. I'd get calls from the White Citizen's Council. I'd get calls from the Black Panthers and so forth. All sorts of calls. The Black Panthers here in Mobile. They even told me that my phone was tapped. That's what I was told. It wasn't a game for me. I was just careful about what I said on the telephone. Of course, I don't know if it was really tapped or not. It was a challenge; it kept you on your toes.

This was over such a long period of time that when it finally was accepted we had progressed along, so many lives had progressed, so that it wasn't that big of a change. Then all the blacks wouldn't come here because they knew we were a white hospital. They themselves wouldn't come here, so we didn't get a very big black population.

The physicians had a special relationship back in the pre-forties. They were respected by the entire community; they were looked upon as gods in their own ranks.

CHAPTER 11

Margie Ward Gatti (1925–)

Registered Nurse

Providence Hospital Nursing School 1946

Director of the operating rooms, Providence Hospital and Doctors Hospital

Interviewed in 1995 at 70 years old

I was born right up the street from the Mobile Infirmary—1925. They torn my birthplace down. I was born up here in a house either the second or third house from the corner on Louiselle. It used to be a Dr. Seller's office. I was born there. That was my uncle's house. My daddy built Dr. Claude Brown's office. I was there 'till I was six. I started to Old Shell Road School and used to walk across St. Mary's Lane and down across the creek and up that way. So you see my whole life has been in Mobile. I trained in the Old Providence Hospital, which was right there on Springhill Avenue. So it's just been in this little circle.

Then the Depression hit and he traded this place for a place on Navco Road. A little acreage; a long way away. When I was born, as soon as Dr. Brown's office was built, we moved in. When we lived on Navco I went to Mertz School, a country school. Then I went to Murphy High School.

I've always wanted to be a nurse. Well, come to find out since I've done all my family research there are five or six of my grandmothers and great-grandmothers that were licensed midwives. Isn't that something? Well see,

I didn't realize it. My daddy didn't want me to be a nurse. He discouraged it. I may be wrong, but there was a time when nurses were just sort of elevated streetwalkers.

He thought a schoolteacher was okay. I think that's what he saw, and he thought a secretary was the elite. I wasn't old enough when I got out of high school to go in training. So I worked a year. One summer I was enrolled in the Hufsteders Business College. I said I'd do it for him, but I knew it was not going to work. I'm just not oriented that way. I started training at the Providence Hospital Nursing School in '43 I think it was. I graduated in '46 at 20.

You lived in the dorms. We had a fairly big class. A little bit better than 20. We studied everything, except you didn't have any management courses per se and you didn't have organizational structure, but you had the basic nursing things. You had anatomy, microbiology, chemistry, and all of that. This was during the war. I was a good student and able to choose to stay here or get more training at Charity, in New Orleans. I got one month contagion (communicable diseases) and six months in surgery. That's where I met Dr. DeBakey and Dr. Balovich. There was a shortage of nurses because of the war. They kept the contagious cases in a separate building—three or four floors. There was no orientation—just get in there and go to it. There was no one to work with you. There was no report—you just walked in, picked up the ball, and went! There wasn't anyone to report to when your shift was over—never saw anyone replace me—just leave when your time's done. I'm telling you, I prayed to get through it a lot.

I remember on the top floor was where the venereal disease cases were. Men—big men—and babies with gonorrhea. There was one little boy recuperating from typhoid fever. Couldn't have been but three or four years old. He was beautiful—milk chocolate skin, those great big eyes. He'd watch from his crib bed as I walked past. One day I came in and found him standing at the elevator. I said, what are you doing here? He opened his mouth and just howled, "I wanna go home!" And he had a jewel like tear just down from his eye. I just held him in my arms and said, "So do I!" Cause I was scared to death. And we stayed there holding on to each other, crying. He didn't want to be there anymore and I wanted to get out too!

During the war, we didn't have, I can only speak for Providence Hospital, a whole lot of doctors. The Muscats (Joe and Vincent) were here. Joe taught the anatomy to the nurses. We were affiliated with Springhill College and he taught anatomy, the growth, and Father Yancy taught the microscopic. We were bussed out to Springhill for the college part. We had Muscat and old Dr. Armstead was there, Dr. Doehring was there, he did the babies. And Dr. Wilson who was, see a long time ago . . . you had your "kingpins." Frazier was in the service at that time. John Wilson was the big boy at Providence. He pulled from all over the state and everything. Whatever he said went. He had his own nurse. Our operating room, to start out, we had two and then one little minor room, I mean just like a closet. And anyway on his days he'd just go back and forth and operate. There wouldn't be anybody else there. Nobody operated that day but him. That's basically a twelve-hour day, but it could go beyond that.

I'll just tell you about the operating rooms, which I remember the best. I can tell you a little bit about the floor. Actually the hospital was basically run by the student nurses. You had the sister who made appearances, and you had a head nurse, and then you had the students. The students were at different levels, like seniors, juniors, freshman, as are still the order. But that was the way it was. It was a prison. That was the way it was. Just, for instance, on a hall like the OB hall and you did three to 11 and you did 11 to seven as a student and you got that in your first year towards the end. There were no graduate nurses on the three to 11 or the 11 to seven. You were there and there was no one else. There wasn't time to—you couldn't stop and chart until the next shift nurse got there and got started. I can remember the OB hall, 45 to 50 patients with just me and an aide. The OB hall had two wings. We had two big wards that had about eight beds in them at the end. But the rest of them were private rooms.

Family members didn't stay at the hospital, not a whole lot. The nurse did most of it. Now the medications weren't as heavy, but you still had to give all the medication, you still did the p.m. care, the back rub; you had to do all that, then you served all the food trays. They would bring them up to us. We served them and then picked them up. But I can remember that OB floor.

That—of course it was a happy floor—at 8:30 p.m., the end of visiting hours, all the lights would come on and you had to do the perineal care where you put them on the pan and washed them with a solution and dried them off with the sponges and all that and take all those bedpans away. The hopper was at the far end of the hall. The hopper, this is gross. It's gross. The hopper was about this big around: it was huge and it was about this high. It was a flush thing and you stepped on it and it was supposed to act like a toilet and suck it down. Supposed to? But it never did. It was always clogged up because of all those little cotton swabs and balls. Then you had the bedpan washer that was in there that you put it in and slammed the door and pulled it shut. But it didn't work real well either, so you had to do a manual swishing around. You couldn't hang around because all the lights were off. Do you see what I'm saying? Get the picture?

One time I came out of a ward with five of them stacked: five bed trays going to the hopper. The hopper was all the way down the hall and around the corner. The linoleum floors were highly waxed. They got away from me! I had to clean all that up. I'm just telling you how it was.

Basically, the head nurse did not do any hands-on. She administrated per floor. On occasion there may be another RN, but many times it was the head nurse and then the sister, she buzzed in and out in between prayers and things like that. They didn't do any work, the sisters didn't. Then there were the students on each floor. And when I was a student you had to pay for everything you broke. Like all the syringes were glass. Yes, and the big 50-cc syringes, they were not cheap. They would count the syringes just before she brought the needles and redid all that. I don't want to get bogged down in all that.

Giving a shot was so different. You used an alcohol lamp, 'bout this big, had a screw top on it and a wick. Over that was this thing, like a little spoon on top. You filled that little spoon with water and lit the lamp to boil the water in it. Then you put the needle in it to sterilize it. You'd put the needle on the syringe. Say the narcotic came in a tablet. You'd put the tablet in the syringe and draw up the water from the spoon to dissolve the narcotic. That was before we had pre-bottled water. But do you see what I'm saying here? The water was used twice! And we didn't have as much infection as patients have today with everything sterilized!

The patients did more or less like they were told. It was accepted. We were the authorities of knowledge and they expected us to do right by them. They trusted us. A lot of healing, well, a lot of it is faith in other people's skills . . . Yeah, I feel that. Most people will heal if they believe that they are getting good care or that they trust the people that are caring for them. And they were getting good care, according to the standards of the day. I mean I'm sure it was the same in all the hospitals. In fact, many may have been better in a smaller town. Much better.

In the operating room there were five student nurses, there was a head nurse, and another graduate who did circulate some and did not do the scrubbing part. They did not take calls, the RNs. The head nurse and the graduates did not take calls. Call was taken by the students. It was set up by ranks. The senior students, they would do the circulating, and the others would do the scrubbing and we stayed in a place upstairs on the roof called the penthouse. That's exactly what it was, it was a little room. It wasn't even screened; had two doors, had bunk beds, and you slept up there. That was it and it was on the roof. And if something came up, then the night supervisor most of the time just hollered up to wake you up. You came down and opened up the operating room and started it. Once in a while she'd come through the OR to be sure everything was moving along. And to see if you were doing the real thing.

We learned by doing. All supplies and the method of sterilization has totally changed. Our water was in tanks. We had a big room with two water tanks that were lit by gas and when it got up to a certain temperature then it was time to fill the tanks and run them. There was no filtering. It was just water out of the tap that you boiled. We lighted it and got the fire up in the thing until it got up to the right temperature and then you timed it the given length of time. This is just the water that you used. At first, we didn't use saline.

Water explodes the cells because it is not isotonic. The only time they use water now is distilled water. Like if you've got cancer, they irrigate with it to blow off the cancer cells. But they normally irrigate now with saline, which is isotonic, it is compatible. Isotonic solution will permeate the cells without exploding it. If it's too low or too high in salt, you've got a problem. If you don't have any salt at all, then it explodes.

The way you collected the water was you had a metal pitcher. The water, you had to take it to the table. So, we had metal pitchers and we had a little kerchief, a little triangular piece of cloth, that we tied and pinned and made a little cover and run that in the autoclave. You use your sterile pitcher, which, actually, it was only sterile when it first came out. But you're talking about people getting well: I'm just telling you what went on and people lived. We didn't kill anybody. So, you just lifted your little flap and filled it up and put your little flap down. That was your water pitchers.

Well, the sterilizer, we had an autoclave for linen, but we didn't do the instruments in with the linen. We had a huge tin that we had water in. It was steel, but it was big and it had a pedal that you pushed down. When you pushed down it opened. The lid came up and the tray came up. When you let loose, the tray went down, submerged, and the lid came down and then it boiled. Once it started boiling—and you would leave it boiling all day to keep it hot. When it started boiling, then you would time your instruments. Then, when they were ready, you raised it and then you picked it up with two towels and you carried them out of that room and down the hall and set them down. You didn't physically touch them except with the towels and then the girl in her gloves and all, she would do that.

After, when they came out with all the blood and crud, then we didn't have instrument washers, they would be physically washed, like knives and forks. They were reused until the end of the day and then they were put up. You grouped them like you separate your silver. That was the instruments.

The linen was folded. We had a laundry in Providence Hospital, in-house laundry. And it would come up to the floor. And we did have a woman that would have been in what we call the linen room and she would fold the sheets and make the sacks. Then they were running autoclaves, which was steam, but I mean it was all fired up and had to get the steam up and let the steam run like that.

I'll tell you something funny. The pilot to the gas was out on this roof where nurses lived when on call. Only this was at the other end. We lived in the middle and this was on the other end of the wing. You could go out and see Springhill. In fact we had windows in the operating room and you could sit in the window and watch the traffic. So did the old Mobile Infirmary. But anyway, when the certain wind from the north would come around, it would blow out the pilot. So we would have to light the pilot. It had a switch in there that you were supposed to turn off the gas, give it a certain amount of time and then go light it. Well, we had this girl; I was her senior, actually we were in the same class, but I had been there longer then she. And she really didn't like to take orders from me. Anyway, she didn't listen and I didn't know this and we were real busy. At the end of the hall in the old Providence, you had some steps and they went to the roof and then there were two doors. Actually, it was glass doors, like French doors, and two screen doors. So in the summertime you had the screen.

Well, Kathleen; I was coming down the hall to get something or other and I couldn't find Kathleen. And she appeared at these doors on the roof and she came staggering through the opening. She was black and she didn't have any eyebrows! I laughed so hard. She looked at me and said, "I've been gassed!" Well, if it hadn't been for the wall around the roof, she would have been blown over. She didn't turn it off. She went out there and stuck that and it blew her up against the wall! But that just shows you some of the things that we had to do.

And the sponges and gloves were reused. Rewashed and reused. Gloves were latex. They had a thing like a laundry thing—form—that only had fingers and you stuck them on there and you clamped them. When they got dry, then you would check them for holes. Then you powdered them and then you put them in the envelopes and then you sterilize them. But you had to wash them first. You reuse that glove and you reuse the gauze sponges. You washed them. I'm just telling you about the spread of disease. We didn't wear gloves.

I'm just saying that we lived through all this. We washed all these organisms, we did all of this and now in the operating room you have infection. Not only that, you have two or three suctions that you use. Then it's the bloodless kind because you are using the cautery. The only time—we had two old portable suctions. And the only way you used them in tonsils, and I'll tell you about tonsils in a minute. You used them if you had a belly full of fluid. And if you knew it ahead of time, you'd have it in there, and if not they'd holler and you'd have to run get it and hope it would work. Roll it in the room and hook it up. And the cautery, they just didn't use that. The only cautery we had was what we called hot cautery. The little box that you used to tie or to cut gut like open up a colostomy. You probed it directly and the current went through this box and made it red-hot and you would comb the cervix with a red-hot poker–like thing. But we didn't have the other things that they use now each day.

There was nobody at that time in Mobile that was formally trained in anesthesia. It was done by nurse anesthetists. They dripped ether or did Pentothal. Nobody was tubed with an intubation. See, Mudd, Dr. DeBakey, and I went over to Charity Hospital for six months. I met DeBakey and Balovich and all of them there. We traveled around the area when other hospitals needed us. Anyway, we—up in Evergreen their lightbulb had burned out and they substituted a sunlamp bulb, which was infrared. It was not a good light, plus it was hot. This was a bad case. It was a gallblad-der with a common duct, which is real hard to beat. But you see, DeBakey wouldn't fuss out of town. You know, he was very good out of town, and we finally managed to do it. I was just saying how different it was. Oh, he wouldn't say anything about that—wouldn't fuss. He wanted to keep friends with me cause I was the only one up there to help him!

Dr. Patton used to fly in. See Dr. Patton was the first neurosurgeon that came in and he was up at Birmingham. Now he wasn't here, this was after the war, because he was in England. Two things that I want to tell you about Dr. Patton. Oh, he was something else! He was a genius, but you could not control him. Anywhere. His wives couldn't control him, nobody could control him. Anyway he came to our hospital. They called him because they had this head injury. I think it was an aneurysm. It was posterior. We went in back here—back of the skull. In the old operating room, we had skylights. Besides windows they had skylights. In brain surgery you not only have to have light, but you got to go in a very small hole. We were in there and I was scrubbed and I had this orderly, Mott Gray, who was a man of all trades. And Mott was doing my circulating, cause it was after hours. Willie, that was Dr. Patton's nickname, Willie didn't come to us to do the case until after everybody else had gone.

But anyway, he was down at a very crucial stage during the surgery and he couldn't see. Well, I dropped out and took Mott and we went up on the roof and put blankets over the skylight and put bricks to darken it. Then we came back and I scrubbed up and went in on the case and Mott took the old drinking cups that used to come in a long thing with a point like a cone. Mott, this is how ingenious Mott was: Mott took that cup, put it over the flashlight, and cut the little thing out to beam in, and then Mott stood right behind him and beamed in and we were able to do the case. I'm telling you this is the truth. We did the case.

Then another time with Willie, now I don't know exactly the date of it, but they built a colored hospital out near Washington Avenue. Willie got a call, this was an aneurysm. They had a nice building but they knew nothing about it. So Willie come and asked me would I go with him and I said yes. So I gathered up stuff. Providence let me go. I went out and got it all set up. It was probably after hours. Everything was after hours, you know, after you did your job then you could do it. I scrubbed up and we were in there and we were operating and he had this flap off as we were working away and the thing burst. And all this blood just welled up. Willie just took, God was with him, just took a hemostat, which you normally don't do in the brain, and he just went in there and clamped it. He got it. He just blindly treated it and we got it and suctioned it out. Then he got a clip in there and everything went fine. But that gives you an idea of what it was like.

You just did it. But you see how these people lived. Just like these people that had the anesthesia with no tubes: no endotracheal tubes, no control of anesthesia. And sometimes they'd raise up off the table and you'd just give them a little bit more. You flew by the seat of your pants. We was doing a disk on this priest one time in the face-down position and he literally raised up on his knees and . . . he was "light." Oh yes, and they had to give him some more. We stopped until they got him down again.

Let me tell you this. This is really funny. I wasn't a student this time. I was running the operating room. This Dr. Wilson I was telling you about, he did a lot of thyroids probably what needed and didn't need to be doctored. Well, Dr. Wilson was the thyroid king. And he did them under local. He would knock them out a little bit under drugs and stuff and then they gave them Pentothal in the vein and put you in "never-never land." The local would be in a flask and it was three-fourths percent Novocaine and a little rubber tube went down in it with a filter and then they had a self-feeding glass syringe, he'd suck it up and down and he'd inject it all around the neck.

One day, it was summer cause we had the windows open, and it was in the south room. He went to the south room—it was the biggest room. We were in the south room working and he did them in sort of a sitting position and he would inject and then they got quiet and they'd give them a little Pentothal and he'd start operating. Then if it wore off, then he'd inject a little more and tell Ms. Rice, who was one of the first anesthetists here, a big lady. Ms. Rice would give them a little more Pentothal. And Wilson, when the patient would complain or something, he'd say, "All right, all right, a little more soothing syrup," and he'd squirt in. This would go on during the cases constantly.

I'm giving you the picture. This had gone on, "All right, all right, a little more soothing syrup." So we were working away and all of the sudden there was a big wreck out there at Springhill Avenue at the light. There was a big, big crash and the car went through the stone wall there at the park. You've never heard anything like it! And Dr. Wilson says, "All right, all right, a little more soothing syrup." He was just set on automatic, see! I thought he was a character and I just cracked up. He was geared to noise, see. That's what he was looking for, the sound. And he just automatically said it, and he went ahead and did his little thing.

Let me tell you this, just to make you laugh, because it was so funny. I don't know whether you have ever been around nuns very much or not. I was Baptist. That was another thing why Daddy didn't want me to go in nursing. It was like I was going into the nunnery—or hell—for my life, you know. I mean, you know you won't get attacked going to a Catholic institution. Well, I was told it was the best nursing school, so anyway. Well the nuns always had some little girls ass-kissing, just right after them, all over the place. Anyway, they would trot behind them and get good grades and get special favors and now and then they would go off to the nunnery. They were looking for recruits to join the nunnery, see.

Anyway, we had this one that they said she had a kidney stone. Well, now I was circulating and we had it all set up. Dr. Boudreau was doing that and I think Dr. Wood was there. Dr. Boudreau was the kidney guy, urologist, and he would just sweat profusely. I mean just gallons. And he had a limp. He was very nice and very competent. We didn't have any AC, so during the summertime we had the windows open and we had these giant fans about this big around that stood up on stands. And once you got your case going, then you moved the fan in position. I mean, the worst thing in the world technically is humidity and sand and bugs. But see, these patients did all right. Then after you got everybody going and it was all draped and everything, then you moved the fan into position to cool Dr Boudreau.

By that time Boudreau was already drenched, he was trying to mop and all that. Well, with this girl, anyway the whole armada of nuns was up there, and they were wearing the big blue hat. You know the dirty wool habits and the big hats that we couldn't get around. And they were in there in the OR and peering, trying to see what he was doing and all. And they were just purple with the heat. It burned me up that they were up there to start with and I couldn't do my job. Couldn't get around them. But they came in like they were sterile, holy and sterile. And you know it just didn't work.

I was getting ready to move the fan up and I got it to the door and Dr. Boudreau said could I get it a little closer. Of course, with all those bodies in there it was right tight. So I gave it a push, you hold it and push the base with your foot. It was tile floors, to get it close. Well, when I did, I got it right up almost to the foot of the table. I didn't touch anything, but I got it up close. The screw that held the fan came out and I didn't know it and of course that fan when I turned it on—it was whirring. It jumped off and went around that table. You've never seen nuns scatter! By God, they grabbed their skirts and they were running! It was the funniest thing that you've ever saw and then it got stuck up under the skirt. I grabbed the cord and unplugged it and got everything loose and took it on out and went and got the other fan. But can you imagine? Can you imagine! We scattered them. Honey, they got out of there! They really did.

I've run an operating room for about 47 years! Then I transferred to Doctors Hospital. I was there at Providence 16 years and moved to Doctors. They came over and asked me to start that. They came to me. Dr. Yem was one of the main ones that, they came to my house and asked me would I take it. Of course, the nuns had not done me right and I went to Doctors because they did not do me right. I had run that operating room over there for 16 years and taught those students, plus the falling, the hole and coming. All of that totally dedicated. Now I'm serious: ours was the very best. Focus on the goal and do it to the very best. I found out that they were hiring new nurses for about two hundred dollars more than I was making as the head of the department. That was before there was control of our salary. They did whatever they wanted to. So, I was offered this job and at that time the money sounded really good and was so much more than I was making. And do you know I was gone a month or two before the head sister knew I wasn't there? That just shows you what they care for you. And I went there and I started there. You know, you need to wake up to reality.

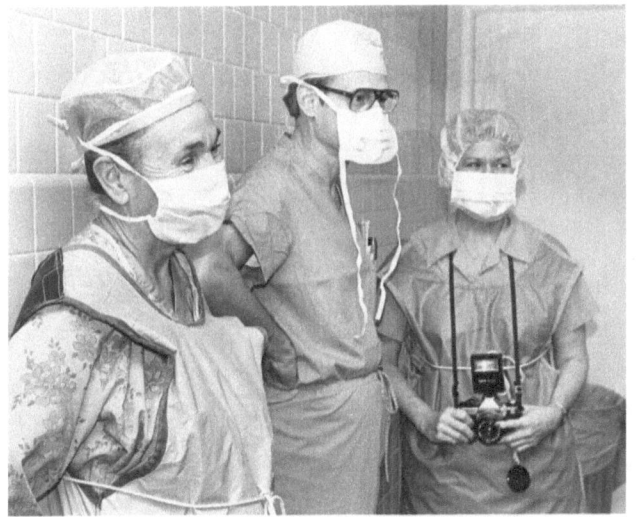

Margi Gatti, RN, and two unnamed professionals in one of the Providence Hospital operating rooms (undated photo)

Providence Hospital: oh, that's another story too. We had to move out. They were going to build the new Providence on Springhill—on the face of the old hospital—when I was in charge of the operating rooms. They were out front digging holes and driving pilots and you could hear it and watch it while you were working. Well in the dead of night, I got a call: our old Providence had split. There was big cracks: all the way, the whole building. Due to the fact, the hole and pounding, the structure was declared unsafe and we had to evacuate.

So they moved all the patients they had, either sent them home or sent them to other hospitals. The prime thing was not to close the hospital. Because Dr. Wood said it was very difficult to close the hospital. So we were going into temporary quarters somewhere. They had a week before we finally moved where they were scouting the areas. Well, they scouted out at Brookley Field. I forget where else they looked. In the interim, we had nothing to do and Mobile Infirmary had picked up our load. So I went down there and worked a week in the operating room to help them and yes, to keep busy.

They finally decided where they would go would be to the old Allen Memorial. Which was the other side of the hospital. It's on Catherine, by the park, next to that nursing home. It was a children's orphanage and upstairs it was a place for unwed mothers, like Florence Crittenden Home. They did the deliveries and things. But it was Daughters of Charity, see, and so was Providence. They made the deal. That was an eye-opener there. Both Daughters of Charity and they agreed to let us have the lower floor and the second floor. The second floor there was rooms and a delivery room. They put the kids on the third floor. Well, when we got ready to move, our top nun told me to go in and survey it and take whatever I needed. One particular thing I had asked for: out in the ward I asked a nun about one room and she said that she really needed that for storage. I told Sister, she said you go in and take it. So you could see the love between the two girls.

What we did, this is interesting, the part that was given to me was the kids' dining room to the back. It was big, and then their playroom, which was another big room across the hall and had windows all around. Then they had a little kitchen. Well, I took the one to the back and put up a partition just halfway where you couldn't see over it. Partitioned that and put some fans up there and made two rooms. Then we had this other room for minor stuff. Across the hall, I made that an equipment room: we had our gas machines and all that stored there. The kitchen I made my sterilizing room. I moved my water tanks in there and my sterilizer in there and then I put the autoclave in the laundry, which was down the hall. So that was my operating room and I worked there for a year and a half to two years.

When they finished the main building, I set up that new operating room at night. When I got through, I had ordered all the instruments, got the linen. I had it all fixed and in place so that when we closed this temporary facility and then I orientated all my people so they would know exactly where everything was and everything was labeled. I washed down all the walls. I had one woman that helped me. Anyway, we closed here one evening, and we opened up the next morning and didn't miss a trick. It can be done if you lay it off; if you planned it and orientate the people. So that's how we would move back in there. We were out of there a year and a half to two years. That was just the starting of the new building. They had to finish the whole building. So we carried on and kept that going.

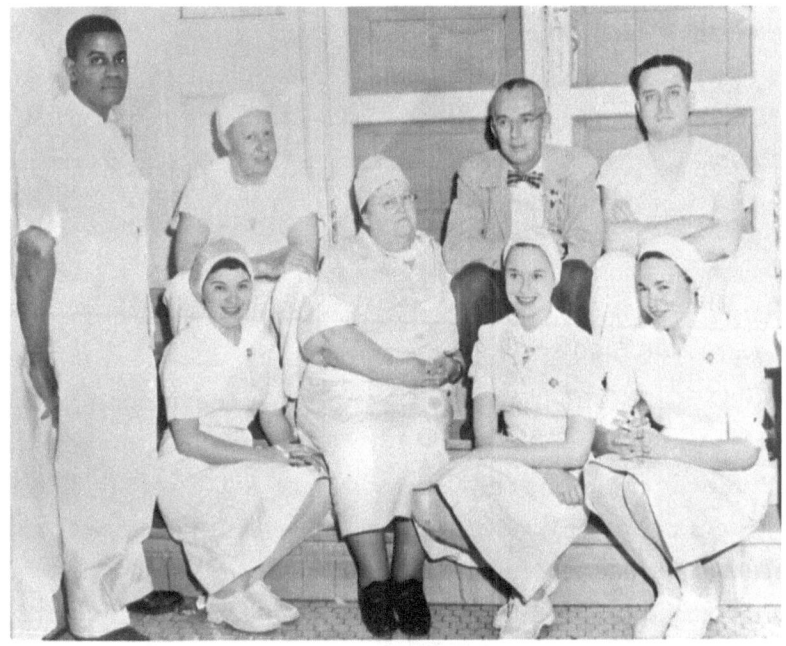

An operating room team at Providence Hospital: (left to right) Mott Gray, orderly, (back row) Dr. Arthur Wood, Vera Rice, CRNA. The others are unidentified (undated photo).

I got married. I was married about a year before I came to Doctors Hospital. I was married for ten years and did the operating rooms. I've done the operating rooms for 47 years. Out of that, ten years I was married. Well, it was interesting. It was a learning experience. It was a learning experience in both areas. Let us say that. In the meantime, I did teach the students. I was like the clinical instructor. No extra pay, no nothing. I had to develop my own books because there was nothing on the market. Since then, a lot of stuff has developed. But at that time, thank God to my training at Charity Hospital, I was able to do that. That gave me the background that I needed.

The strongest influence on medicine was insurance. All results have stemmed from this and it is still protected. The war ended and more younger docs come back to Mobile, and some specialists come with them. Soon, the docs have more and more time off with all these fellows being in town together. Then the patient is not seeing the same physician all the time and the relationship suffers. There was a period of time, of course, where you were encouraged to go to the hospital for everything, for a hang-nail. So that's what they did. They did that and they raped that insurance availability. Then when that was raped, then they got into the outpatient thing, and then that started booming.

Then offices competed because they stopped them from going to the hospitals, so that opened up a place for them to make all their money with their clinics fully staffed. That's right. And what you did there instead of controlling it in such a way that it was part of the hospital to be in the hospital environment so that you had access to everything that you needed. They had their clinics and the freestanding and that divorced the hospital from the physician. He divorced the hospital and left the hospital with the full financial burden too. And up until that point in time the hospital had taken the financial burden for everything. They had all the labs, they had it three or four hours staffed. Everything that hospital had and the hospital catered to the physician. He was gone. And everything circled around him and he pulled out and left them high and dry . . . still in a deadlock here and insurance is sitting out here controlling the puppets.

My personal opinion is that there are very few people who will stand by you when the real crunch comes. Dr. DeBakey and I used to talk about it and you can count them on one hand. If you've got that many, you're doing damn good. You've got to face reality and not let; you've got to know the score and do your thing and be over it and go on through this journey. That's a fact. Accept that fact and don't let it pull you down. Because if it does, you cannot be productive. You just have to wipe that out. You do it for your own self-satisfaction and nobody else. That's the only thing. That is the only thing that really means something to me.

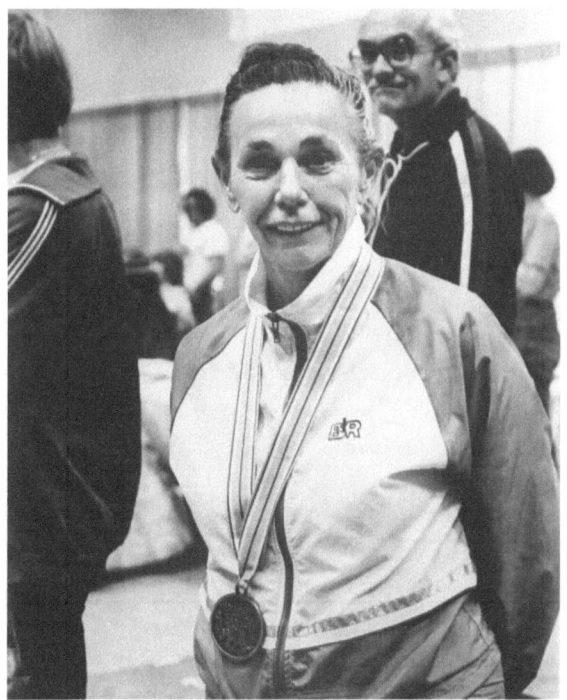

M. Gatti, RN (undated photo)

When I talk to my God and he looks at me, I hope he says job well done. I hope. And that's all I really want. Whatever, I've give it my best shot. That's right. You know we didn't ask to come here and we ain't going to ask to go. We were equal, we were comrades. Oh yeah, and worked hard, played hard. The best parties you ever saw. You know just marvelous and we all loved each other. There was a kinship there. And it's still there.

CHAPTER 1 REFERENCES

J Asplund. "Birth of the Blues." *AHA News*, 2/23/98, v34 (7).

R Ball. "What Medicare's Architects Had in Mind." *Health Affairs*, Winter 1995, v14(4).

EH Beardsley. *A History of Neglect: Health Care for Blacks and Mill Workers in the Twentieth-Century South*. Knoxville: The University of Tennessee Press, 1986.

EH Beardsley. "Desegregating Southern Medicine 1945–1970." *International Social Science Review*, 2001, v71(1 and 2).

HK Beecher, MD Altschule. *Medicine at Harvard: The First Three Hundred Years*. Hanover, NH: University Press of New England, 1977.

PB Beeson. "The Natural History of Medical Subspecialties." *Annals of Internal Medicine*, 1980: 93.

J Bordley, AM Harvey. *Two Centuries of American Medicine 1776–1976*. Philadelphia: WB Saunders Company, 1976.

K Dawley. "Origins of Nurse-Midwifery in the United States and Its Expansion in the 1940s." *Journal of Midwifery & Women's Health*, Mar.–Apr. 2003, v48(2).

J Duffy. *The Healers: A History of American Medicine*. Urbana and Chicago: University of Illinois Press, 1976.

GQ Flynn. "American Medicine and Selective Service in World War II." *The Journal of the History of Medicine and Allied Sciences*, 1987, v42 (3).

M Galdston. "Ambulance Notes of a Bellevue Hospital Intern: May 1938." *Journal of Urban Health*, Dec. 1999, v76(4).

KM Gerber. H&HN—Eight Decades of Health Care: 80th Anniversary. The 1950s. *Hospitals and Health Networks/AHA*, Apr. 2007, v81(4).

RVN Ginn. *The History of the US Army Medical Service Corps*. Washington, DC: US Government Printing Office, 1996.

E Ginzberg. "The Shift to Specialism in Medicine: The US Army in World War II." *Academic Medicine*, May 1999, v74(5).

T Hager. "The Saga of a Sulfa Drug Pioneer." *NPR Weekend Edition*, 12/23/2006.

PG Harrison. "Riveters, Volunteers and WACS." In *Down the Years: Articles on Mobile's History*. M. Thomason, editor. Gulf South Historical Review, 2001.

H&HN—Eight Decades of Health Care: 80th Anniversary. The 1930s. *Hospitals and Health Networks/AHA*, Feb. 2007, v81(2): 12–15.

H&HN—Eight Decades of Health Care: 80th Anniversary. The 1940s. *Hospitals and Health Networks/AHA*, Mar. 2007, v81(3).

K Hoyt. "Vaccine Innovation: Lessons from World War II." *Journal of Public Health Policy*, 2006, v27(1).

WP Jones. "Black Workers and the CIOs Turn toward Racial Liberalism: Operation Dixie and the North Carolina Lumber Industry, 1946–1953." *Labor History*, Aug. 2000, v41(3).

CAB Jordan. "Graduate Medical Education in Mobile 1859–1981." *Journal of the Medical Association of the State of Alabama*, Oct. 1981, v51(4): 16,18, 24–29.

BA Lazarus. "The Practice of Medicine and Prejudice in a New England Town: The Founding of Mount Sinai Hospital." *Journal of American Ethnic History*, Spring 1991, v10(3).

DM Little. "The Founding of the Specialty Boards." *Anesthesiology*, Sept. 1981, v155(3).

BK Loftin. "A Social History of the Mid-Gulf South (Panama City–Mobile) 1930–1950." Dissertation, University of Southern Mississippi, Aug. 1971.

LA Mansfield. "Dreaming Big Dreams: The University of Alabama at Birmingham School of Medicine." *Southern Medical Journal*, Aug. 2003, v96(8).

MM McLaurin. "Mobile Blacks and World War II: The Development of a Political Consciousness." *Gulf Coast Politics in the Twentieth Century.* Ted Caragorge, editor. Journal of the Proceedings Gulf Coast History and Humanities Conference, 1972, v4.

Mobile Press, "Medicare Fight Won by Hospital," 2/23/67.

N Moiden. "Evolution of Leadership in Nursing: Nodeem Moiden Looks at Leadership Style and Theory and Relates Developments through History to Leadership in Today's Profession." *Nursing Management*, Jan. 2002, v9(7).

B Nelson. "Organized Labor and the Struggle for Black Equality in Mobile during World War II." *The Journal of American History*, Dec. 1993, v80(3): 952–88.

Newsweek. "Medicine's Great Journey, One Hundred Years of Healing," Nov. 9, 1992, v120(19).

MC O'Brien. "Prehospital Care—An Historical Perspective." *Trauma Quarterly*, 1998, v14(2).

SM Reverby. *Ordered to Care: The Dilemma of American Nursing, 1850–1945.* Cambridge, MA: Cambridge University Press, 1987.

PP Reynolds. "Public Health Then and Now: Dr. Louis T. Wright and the NAACP: Pioneers in Hospital Racial Integration." *American Journal of Public Health*, June 2000, v90(6).

S Roberds. "Roberds Named New Nursing Vice President." *Mobile Infirmary Medical Center Tempo Magazine*, Nov./Dec. 1984.

WG Rothstein. *American Medical Schools and the Practice of Medicine: A History*. New York: Oxford University Press, 1987.

JW Schrock. "Lifelong Learning." *Emergency Medicine Clinics of North America*. Aug. 2006, v24(3).

LA Scofea. "The Development and Growth of Employer-Provided Health Insurance." *Monthly Labor Review*, Mar. 1994, v117(3).

DB Smith. *Health Care Divided: Race and Healing a Nation*. Ann Arbor, MI: University of Michigan Press, 1998.

MC Smith, LJ Holmes. *Listen to Me Good: The Life Story of an Alabama Midwife*. Columbus: Ohio State University Press, 1996.

L Sokoloff. "The Rise and Decline of the Jewish Quota in Medical School Admissions." *Bulletin of the New York Academy of Medicine*, Nov. 1992, v68(4).

R Stevens. "Issues for American Internal Medicine through the Last Century." *Annals of Internal Medicine*, Oct. 1986, v105(4).

TP Wasley. "Health Care in the Twentieth Century: A History of Government Interference and Protection." *Business Economics*, Apr. 1933, v28(2).

Wikipedia. "History of Mobile, Alabama." http://en.wikipedia.org/wiki/History_of_Mobile,_Alabama

H Wiseman. "Graduate Medical Education in Mobile." *Journal of the Medical Association of the State of Alabama*, Feb. 1983, v52(8): 43–49.

G Whorton. "Regulations for Student Nurses in 1940." *RN*, Oct. 1997, v60(10).